How *to* Get Out *of the* Hospital Alive

How *to* Get Out *of the* Hospital Alive

A GUIDE TO PATIENT POWER

SHELDON P. BLAU, M.D., F.A.C.P., F.A.C.R.
and ELAINE FANTLE SHIMBERG

MACMILLAN · USA

MACMILLAN
A Simon & Schuster Macmillan Company
1633 Broadway
New York, New York 10019

Library of Congress Cataloging-in-Publication Data

Blau, Sheldon Paul, 1935–

How to get out of the hospital alive: a guide to patient power / by Sheldon
  P. Blau and Elaine Fantle Shimberg.
    p.   cm.
    Includes bibliographical references and index.
    ISBN 0-02-862363-0
    1. Hospital patients.   2. Hospital care.   3. Patient education.
I. Shimberg, Elaine Fantle, 1937– .   II. Title.
RA965.6.B56   1997
362.1' 1—dc32   96-29504
                                                                 CIP

DESIGN BY KEVIN HANEK

10 9 8 7 6 5 4 3 2 1

Printed in the United States of America

Chapter 5

"What Parents Need to Know" is from *For Healthcare Professionals: Guidelines on Prevention and Response to Infant Abductions* by John B. Rabun, Jr., ACSW, and reprinted with permission of the National Center for Missing and Exploited Children (NCMEC). Copyright © NCMEC 1989, 1991, 1992, 1993, and 1996. All rights reserved.

Chapter 6

"A Patient's Bill of Rights" reprinted with permission of the American Hospital Association, copyright © 1992.

"What You Can Do" *from People's Medical Society Newsletter,* June 1996, vol. 15, no. 3.

"An Open Book" excerpted from the September 1995 issue of the *Harvard Health Letter,* copyright © 1995, President and Fellows of Harvard College.

Chapter 7

"Perseveration of Laboratory Test Ordering: A Syndrome of Affecting Clinicians," from *Journal of the American Medical Association* 249 (4 February 1983): 639. Copyright © 1983, American Medical Association.

Chapter 8

"Your Life in My Hands" reprinted courtesy of *American Health,* copyright © 1995 by Dr. Andrew G. Kadar.

Disclaimer

This book has been written to help advise patients on how they can become more involved in making informed decisions about their own medical care. As each person is unique in his or her physical and emotional makeup, this book does not presume to replace the need to communicate and work with a competent personal physician. It is intended in no way to replace professional medical care.

This book is dedicated
to Bette, who saved
my life and is my life
— *S.P.B.*

and to Barbara,
who did it her way
— *E.F.S.*

"Primum, non nocere"

First, do no harm.

— HIPPOCRATIC OATH

Contents

Acknowledgments

The authors are indebted to a number of people, both lay and health-care professionals, who shared with us their time and their personal stories of hospital experiences.

We especially thank our spouses, Bette Blau and Hinks Shimberg, who supported our efforts in many ways, including helping to ferret out additional anecdotes from people with whom they were in contact. We also owe a tremendous debt of appreciation and thanks to our agent, Faith Hamlin.

Special thanks also to Richard Hodes, M.D.; Bonnie S. Michelman, CHPA, CPP; Chuck Figaro; Andrew Malbin, M.D.; Murray Canter, M.D.; The Tampa Hillsborough County Public Library; The Boston Public Library; Mark A. Hart; Scott M. Chase, D.O.; Roger Goodman; and Lane France, M.D.

For their help, support, and devotion, special thanks to Ashley, Debra, Brett, Steven, Vicki, Butch, Mark Goodman, M.D., Lou, Jim, Peggy, Jonathan Bush, Chuck Hyman, and Marty Bond.

A particularly warm thank you to our children who, through their advice, guidance, and humor, helped us make this book happen.

Introduction

In that delicate parchment-thin fragment of time between sleep and wakening, I questioned why a horse was sitting on my chest. He's too heavy, I concluded. I can't breathe with him sitting there. Once fully awake I realized, of course, that there was no horse. There still was, however, a tightening—like a band across my chest.

I'm a board-certified doctor of internal medicine and a rheumatologist. I spent years being trained to analyze symptoms and determine a diagnosis and have been in practice more than thirty years. Nevertheless, I immediately told myself I was suffering only from indigestion and heartburn and headed to the medicine cabinet to find some antacid.

Popping a tablet into my mouth, I flipped on the television. It was January 17, 1994. The news channel reporter was describing a 6.4 earthquake that had hit Los Angeles. Both of my children, my son-in-law, and my only grandchild live there. I sank into a chair, my eyes never leaving the TV screen. The quake's epicenter, I learned, was about ten or twenty miles from my daughter's and granddaughter's home. I popped another antacid into my mouth, crunching it forcefully between my teeth.

My indigestion did not let up. The tightening across my chest continued. I was distracted from the accounts of the quake only by a sudden awareness of the pain moving down my left arm, settling in my wrist. I told myself that if a patient complained of this type of arm pain, I would think it was of rheumatic origin. But I knew it was cardiac.

"I need some coffee," I thought. "I haven't had breakfast." I continued in my denial until the coffee mug dropped from my hand. I stood stupidly for a few seconds, breathless with the pain. Finally I admitted the obvious. I was having a problem with my heart.

I crossed the kitchen to the wall phone, dialed my partner's number, then pulled over a chair so I could sit. When he answered, I rambled on about having had no breakfast, seeing the news about the earthquake, and finally got around to mentioning having some minimal pain in my chest. He was at my door in twenty minutes to drive my wife and me to the emergency room of the very hospital to which I admitted my own patients. I assumed I'd be checked by one of the doctors there and sent home within the hour.

Instead, the ER physician ran an EKG. It was unimpressive, which is medical talk for "normal." Regardless, the doctor suggested I stay a few days for observation. Again, that's medical talk for "I don't think there's anything wrong with you, but I don't want to screw up, so I'll admit you to cover myself if I'm wrong." He did and he was.

I have a family history of angina. My mother had a pacemaker inserted into her chest when she was seventy. My uncle died of heart trouble in his fifties and my brother has heart disease. But I'm the healthy one, I reminded myself. I was just back from a skiing trip. I have a completely outfitted exercise room and usually work out for one to two hours a day. There couldn't be anything wrong with my heart.

The cardiologist wanted to give me heparin, a drug used to thin blood in order to prevent a clot that could cause a stroke or a heart attack. I refused it. I know that heparin can also cause bleeding into the brain. So does he. I'm just more afraid of it than he is. After all, it's my brain.

Then he suggested giving me rat poison. He doesn't call it that, of course. He used the correct name, which is Coumadin. But it's still the leading commercial agent used to kill rats. I said no to the Coumadin as well. Since I refused both the cerebral bleeder and the rat poison, he threw up his hands, muttering something about the difficulty in treating physicians. His next offer was Valium, enough to put me to sleep.

Valium is a tranquilizer. While it didn't quite make me tranquil enough to sleep, it did carry me off to that gray area where the periphery of people and voices blurs. My facial muscles felt as though they were melting as my eyes grew heavy and began sinking into the back of my head. I knew that I was "zonked." My wife thought I was having a stroke and had the neurologist paged.

The neurologist was a resident and not totally sure of what's what, but she felt somewhat confident that it wasn't a stroke. She ordered numerous blood tests, the results of which she never saw, because she was "off duty" when they returned.

I was told that I must remain in the hospital until Monday to have a stress test. Unfortunately, the next day was Sunday. Nothing much gets done in a hospital on Sundays. Stress tests are not done, labs are open only for emergencies, even the clocks seem to slow down. The only thing that didn't slow down was the steady flow of visitors.

My room filled with nervous family members milling around, talking to one another in stage whispers. In my tranquilized state, their whispers seemed more like shouting. "What can we get you?" they asked, peering down into my face like visitors at an aquarium.

"Spareribs," I replied.

There was nervous laughter. I remembered it was Sunday. We always had family dinner on Sunday, so I mumbled to my wife through a mouth that seemed defective that she should order in Italian food to feed this group. My brother offered to pick up the food, taking my credit card with him.

Everyone sat around on chairs and my bed eating Italian food. My mother-in-law complained that the pasta was undercooked. My brother complained they didn't include the extra Parmesan cheese. I opened my mouth to complain about how I felt trying to negotiate—on a biochemical basis—the Valium and pasta.

My heart began fluttering, demonstrating a loss of the regular sinus rhythm of the heart. I felt dizzy. The Valium won and my face flopped into the pasta.

I was in no shape to argue, so I scrawled my signature on a form permitting them to perform an angiogram, a procedure in which dye is injected into the coronary artery, highlighting blocked areas. What I signed could have included my paying off the physicians' mortgages and giving them my firstborn son for all I knew.

If a blockage was severe, an angioplasty would immediately follow. They gave me more Valium to reduce my anxiety. It's hard not to be anxious when you know what's happening to you and what could go wrong. Complications of these procedures included infection, bleeding, and rupture of the coronary artery.

What I feared could go wrong did. A technician jabbed a bore needle into the femoral artery in my groin. It's a large needle. It has to be because a plastic catheter is fed through it and inserted up into the heart. Dye injected into the catheter winds its way into the coronary artery, revealing on a large monitor for all (including me) to see where a blockage might be located. We all saw it.

"You've got an artery that is 90 percent closed," the cardiologist said. "We're going to thread a wire up your aorta, inflate a balloon, and open up that artery." They did so, then checked with the dye to see if progress had been achieved. As the technician was inserting the tubing into my artery, he said suddenly, "Whoops. We ruptured your artery." That's just what they had done—ruptured my coronary artery. I looked at the monitor. Dye was spurting. What next? I thought. But I knew full well. I would need immediate emergency open-heart surgery to repair the damage.

Right before the surgery, I suffered a heart attack. There was bleeding from a blood vessel. Heart tissue, deprived of vital oxygen, died. For six hours, my brain and other Vital organs were nourished with blood circulating through a heart-lung machine. I survived, only to awake in a multi-bed coronary intensive care unit popularly known as the ICCU.

I had tubes in every orifice. I couldn't talk because I had a tube in my trachea. I didn't mind not talking. It was frustrating, but rather comforting. I was alive. I knew that I was alive and that I had been through a death-defying time. I had pain all over and suspected that I must have been hit by a truck, a large one.

The first person I saw was my wife. I could see by the look on her face that she also knew that I had been through a death-defying experience. She told me our grown kids were coming in from California where they both live. Now I *knew* I was in trouble.

I had what resembled a paper zipper on my chest and on my right leg. It didn't occur to me that eight people had removed a vein from my leg, sawed open my breastbone (the sternum), spread my sternum open to gain access to my heart, and then did stuff in my chest.

Since I couldn't talk, I assumed that I had a tube in my trachea with an opening (called a tracheostomy). I knew that if I put my finger over the hole I would be able to speak. With one wobbly hand, I reached for the hole. But there was no hole, no tracheostomy. I just couldn't speak.

A nurse arrived and told me I couldn't speak. As though I didn't know that. I decided I must have had a stroke. She gave me a small blackboard to write my thoughts. I wrote, "I can't talk." She nodded—no big news to her.

It's time for assessment. I said to myself, "I can still think, I can still move, albeit with pain. I can live without talking because I can still write, even though no one but my wife can read my writing."

A respiratory therapist came in. "I'm removing your endotracheal tube," she announced as she released a clamp. I coughed and she pulled out a one-foot-long tube. Now I could speak.

My wife reappeared and told me I was going to be all right. Somehow, despite my precarious position, I believed her. Her nurturing, protective, mothering act worked, giving me faith that all would be okay. While I wasn't 100 percent certain, I was at least 90 percent sure. Being 90 percent certain that you're not going to die leaves you on your toes. That 10 percent uncertainty makes you hyperreact to everything.

The physician's assistant arrived and told me who he was. I didn't want a physician's assistant as long as I was 10 percent certain I might die. I wanted a real doctor—not only a real doctor, but a dozen doctors, all professors, all with gray hair, all super specialists. I asked for my personal doctor, but it was now evening and he wasn't on call. That 10 percent was still in the forefront of my mind. I insisted that he be called, as well as my partners, both of whom are medical doctors. I wanted no mistakes, no judgment calls. I didn't want to die.

The physician's assistant told me that my blood pressure was 90 systolic, too low. He thought I needed a blood transfusion. This was like shooting three dull arrows into me. First, I didn't want him to make the decision to give me blood. Second, I didn't want someone else's blood. I was afraid of AIDS, hepatitis, and an autoimmune reaction due to a mismatch. Lastly, I wanted a second opinion. I called for the surgeon.

The surgeon arrived. He told me that I had already been exposed to fifteen bottles of blood while I was hooked up to the heart-lung machine, so that one more wouldn't make any difference. He assured me that the blood had been tested for HIV. I thought of Arthur Ashe and wondered what they told him.

I insisted that they speak to my partner, who is the best physician I know. After a short delay, I accepted the blood transfusion. They were afraid to give me pain medications because my blood pressure was so low. My sternum had just been sawed open. It was put back and held together with steel sutures. Breathing caused enormous pain. If I coughed, it was like being run over.

The respiratory therapist returned to tell me I must "breathe deeply and cough and have a nice day." She looked about fourteen years old. I could imagine pigtails flying behind her as she hurried out the door.

I looked up at one of the three IVs and read "Levophed" on one of the bottles. It's a peripheral vasoconstrictor and is used to maintain blood pressure. It also stimulates the heart while it dilates the coronary arteries. That's the good news. But this drug must be used with extreme caution. Under certain conditions, Levophed can trigger heart fibrillation, anaphylactic shock, high blood pressure, and respiratory distress. When I was an intern we called Levophed the "dread phed." Or "leave them dead with Levophed." (Interns have sick jokes like that to get them through some of the horrors they must deal with.) I now was convinced I would die. I never saw a patient get off the dread phed.

My wife returned. I pointed to the Levophed bottle. She knew about Levophed. She turned to each patient in the ICCU and saw Levophed in each bottle. She gave me the news; I was convinced we all would die. She knew what I was thinking. After thirty-eight years of marriage, she always knew what I was thinking. She told me with the patience of a mother with a slow child that since all the patients had the dread phed running, they all couldn't die.

She quickly recognized that I would not accept this logic, so she got the heart surgeon and told him what I thought. He assured me that all the patients would not die (only some of them?). He said it was SOP (standard operating procedure) to use Levophed. I believed him. He also knew that I was anxious and ordered the Levophed to be stopped. To me, it was like the warden's last-hour reprieve. I was saved. Levophed was stopped. The execution was halted.

Soon I was transferred out of the ICCU to one of the step-up rooms where there was less intensive care. That meant I should be getting better. But I wasn't. I had shaking chills so severe that I needed extra blankets. My wife, who decided to stay in the hospital day and night, much to the dismay of the nursing staff, suggested that I needed an infectious disease consult. He arrived to tell me that he suspected I had an infectious disease, probably staph, and that an antibiotic called Vancomycin should be begun. This drug must be given intravenously for two weeks. I still had an IV going with heparin, the blood thinner, so it was relatively easy to add another drug in the IV line.

In a few days, it would be very difficult to find a vein (i.e., an easily accessible vein). In a week, it would be impossible. By the time I left the hospital, there would be talk of a "cut down." That meant cutting into the skin in order to reach a less visible vein.

As a result of a paralytic ileus (my intestines stopped their peristaltic activity), more specialists stopped by. Each specialist was afraid of missing something, so many redundant blood tests were performed. My arms began to resemble two salamis. They became black and blue, then purple and swollen. I developed a phlebitis from the caustic nature of the Vancomycin and the repeated venipunctures. I needed and received hot moist soaks. Despite this complication, vampires calling themselves phlebotomists came to draw blood four and five times a day. My wife finally suggested that many of these blood tests could be combined into one venipuncture and the blood letting dropped to twice a day. My arms looked worse. My fingers became swollen stubs.

The next day, the infectious disease specialist triumphantly returned to tell me that the heart catheter had grown staph from its tip. Now what, I wondered, made them culture the tip of the catheter? I was too sick to see the obvious; I was running a high fever and having chills, sure signs of infection.

I soon learned that, unbeknownst to me or my family, staphylococcal disease, a highly contagious, often fatal blood infection, was present in a number of patients throughout the coronary care unit of the hospital. My roommate had a staph empyema (pus) that was being drained into a bottle not more than five feet from my bed. I questioned the wisdom of my being so close to him, having just returned from open-heart surgery and with a fresh wound from my sternum to my abdomen. My heart surgeon agreed and arranged for my transfer to another room.

My new roommate was a man who'd had open-heart surgery six months before. He now had a staphylococcal infection in his sternum (staph osteomyelitis). While not an ideal situation, it was slightly better than what I had before. Besides him, there were two more patients on the ward with a staph infection. One had

Methicillin (an antibiotic) Resistant Staph Aureas (MRSA), a disease I had only heard of but never seen. He would eventually die of this as most patients with MRSA do. The last patient was comatose following open-heart surgery. The doctors theorized that she too had staph in her blood. It was apparent to me that there was staph in many areas of the hospital.

I rationalized when I saw that my heart surgeon had no patients with complicating staphylococcal disease. I told myself, this was not a result of infection from my doctor. He actually looked cleaner than the other doctors I had observed. When he came to visit me after surgery, my friends and family remarked how he almost "shone." I looked at his nails as he examined me. They were, as they should be, ultra-short and clean. I glanced at his nose for pimples—I saw none. I looked into his eyes to judge if they were red, as a person who sneezes a lot might have a chronic conjunctivitis and by this route, spread staph. His eyes were bright—no conjunctivitis. In this Kangaroo Court, I judged the surgeon not guilty.

But I still had a potentially lethal staph infection in my blood that was being treated with an antibiotic that must be given intravenously. It would need to continue even after my discharge from this hospital.

My hospital stay continued to challenge my determination to survive. I realized I was completely at the mercy of the hospital and its staff. It was quite an awakening. During my professional career I had seen thousands of patients and, of necessity, had admitted many patients to various hospitals. But until this point, I had always played the role of doctor, not patient. Now I was learning all too well what it was like to be in the hospital bed, rather than at bedside.

Complications like the ones that happened to me and to others occur daily in hospitals—good hospitals as well as bad and so-so institutions—throughout the country. Fortunately, because I was a physician and also because my wife, who is not afraid to speak up, was with me at all times to intercede on my behalf and to ask questions when I was unable to, I survived my hospital stay. I was released after seventeen days and soon recovered from both the surgery and my ordeal in the hospital. But it got me to thinking.

I don't believe things happen without a reason. There usually is a "plan" behind what we mortals refer to as "coincidence." The more I thought about it, the more I was sure that my unsettling hospital experiences had a purpose: to encourage me to write a book informing others how to remain constantly on guard, to gain patient power, to protect themselves so they could become their own patient advocate. Too many patients worry about exposing their rear ends in skimpy hospital gowns when they should be more concerned about exposing themselves to serious illness and potentially fatal incidents in the hospital.

My cardiologist had told me that my life and how I practiced medicine would change after my heart surgery. He was right. I began to see fewer patients, spent more time with each patient, sent flowers to those people I thought needed a lift, and in general, became a better doctor. The near-death experience also encouraged me to slow down and to smell those proverbial flowers. It also prompted the writing of this book.

Is my hospital experience unique? Unfortunately, it is not. Hospital errors are made daily because they are human errors, made by humans who often may be overworked in understaffed areas, who may be careless, tired, or under the influence of drugs or alcohol. It happened to me and I'm a doctor; it happens to lay patients as well. It could happen to you. Consider these few recent examples:

- A diabetic patient was admitted to the surgical ward of a major hospital to have his right leg amputated. Instead, his left leg was removed.

- A seventy-seven-year-old man died when the respiratory therapist mistook him for another patient and turned off his ventilator.

- A doctor mistook a dialysis catheter in an elderly patient's abdomen for a feeding tube and ordered feeding solution pumped into it. Six days later, the patient died.

- A sixteen-year-old waiting in her hospital room to be taken down to the operating room for an emergency appendectomy was surprised when an aide served her a breakfast tray. Had the teenager eaten it, she could have aspirated the contents of her stomach into her lungs and died of pneumonia.

- A thirty-four-year-old man was returned to his room after a hepatic arteriogram. "Hop up on the bed," the orderly told him cheerfully. Had he done so, the patient could have bled to death from the puncture wound leading from his groin into the hepatic artery.

Sadly, these errors and "near" errors are not rare situations. A recent study conducted to identify and correct situations compromising patient safety in intensive care facilities examined 390 incidents. Of that number, 106 caused "actual" harm and 284 "potential" harm. There was one death, eighty-six severe complications, and eighty-eight complications of minor severity.

Other studies reveal physician errors in which doctors were not adequately trained, demonstrated poor clinical judgment, and showed poor teamwork. Carelessness or incompetence accounted for major errors. Errors even occurred during the seemingly simple act of admitting patients to the hospital. The most prevalent errors uncovered by the study were mistakes made by admissions clerks while inputting the uniform number codes identifying medical services, diagnoses, and procedures by physicians. Nursing staffs made mistakes in the five rules for the correct administration of medication: right patient, right drug, right dose, right route, right time.

Human error is a significant cause of fatalities associated with blood transfusions. In fact, human error in identifying patients or specimens due to fatigue, stress, and lack of attention by technologists, nurses, and physicians can cause routine safety procedures to be circumvented.

Poor communication between patient and staff may account for additional errors. There are, for example, various medications—such as non-steroidal anti-inflammatory drugs like Feldene and Voltaren—that must be stopped one week before surgery to prevent excessive bleeding and possible shock. If the patient isn't asked specifically what medications he or she is presently taking (or if the patient doesn't know or remember), major and sometimes fatal problems can develop.

According to the American Hospital Association, the number of U.S. hospitalizations per year is 33,282,124 (1995 figures). Is being a patient hazardous to one's health? What can be done to protect a patient? What steps can we take to deliver patient power to those of us who must enter a hospital or whose loved ones become patients?

Today, the practice of medicine and the delivery of health care is big business, often impersonal and highly technical. This trilogy of factors is largely responsible for the increase in hospital-caused errors in medication, wrong-sited surgeries, infections, laboratory mistakes, and other hospital horrors. Insurance regulations rather than physician expertise dictate lengths of stays, procedures, and often, actual medication protocols. Capitation, in which a provider is paid a fixed amount regardless of the service rendered, can also negatively affect patient care.

Hospitals, hustling for a greater share of Medicare, Medicaid, HMOs, and PPOs, sock it to the private payer as the golden goose in a procedure known as cost shifting. This means charging privately insured patients more in order to counterbalance underpayment by Medicare and Medicaid, bad debts, and charity work in an (often futile) attempt to lower costs without sacrificing quality of care (or the patient). Patients have become "cases" and "beds filled" rather than retaining their human designations.

Hospital risk management specialists would do well to follow the example of this book: to help educate patients and their families so that they can become knowledgeable patient advocates, to assure them of their right to ask questions, to question procedures, and to become active participants on the healthcare team.

How to Get Out of the Hospital Alive demystifies the hospital bureaucracy by defining it in human terms, describing who does what and why, telling where and how to get the necessary information in order to make informed decisions, and encouraging patients to become empowered even while wearing a hospital gown. It offers accounts of recent medical errors and suggests how they might have been avoided. It explains numerous medical tests, as well as how and why they are performed and how to be certain you are given the procedure and/or medication prescribed for you.

A businessman tells the story of a nurse coming into his hospital room and saying, "I'm here to give you an enema."

He was somewhat surprised as he had been admitted for a knee injury. "Why?" he asked.

"Your doctor ordered it," he was told. Being compliant, the man reluctantly rolled over and submitted to the procedure.

That afternoon, his roommate's doctor stopped by. "How are you feeling?" the physician asked the man in bed two.

The roommate shrugged. "The same."

The doctor looked surprised. "The enema didn't help?" he asked. He had ordered it for his patient, not the businessman.

An elderly Jewish woman was surprised when a young priest came into her semi-private room and proceeded to give her last rites. When he had finished, she said, "That was lovely, Father. I didn't want to interrupt you, but I'm Jewish."

He looked startled and glanced down at the list in his hand. He had been requested to administer to Mrs. Garcia in the other bed.

While these true stories may seem amusing, similar mistakes could prove and have proven deadly.

This book specifies actions patients (and their families) must take before, during, and even after a hospital stay in order to ensure safe and proper treatment, quick and uneventful recovery, and the opportunity to arrive home in better shape than when they left.

Who We Are and Why We Are Writing This Book

DR. SHELDON BLAU received his B.A. from City College of New York in 1957, graduating Phi Beta Kappa. In 1961 he graduated from Albert Einstein College of Medicine and did both his internship and residency in internal medicine at Montefiore Hospital and Medical Center in New York City. In 1965 he completed a fellowship in Rheumatology at Albert Einstein College of Medicine as an N.I.H. fellow. From 1969 to 1990, he was Chief of Rheumatology at Nassau County Medical Center. He presently serves as an attending physician and consultant at numerous hospitals in Long Island and is a Clinical Professor of Medicine at SUNY in Stony Brook, New York. He served on the Board of Professional Conduct of the New York State Department of Health for two terms.

Dr. Blau has written or coauthored more than forty publications for both professional and lay readers on a variety of medical subjects including arthritis in children and the elderly, lupus, and other rheumatologic topics.

ELAINE FANTLE SHIMBERG is the author of fourteen books, including *Living with Tourette Syndrome, Gifts of Time, Depression: What Families Should Know, Strokes: What Families Should Know,* and *Relief from IBS: Irritable Bowel Syndrome,* as well as hundreds of articles published in such newspapers and magazines as *Glamour, Essence, Woman's Day,* and *Reader's Digest.*

She is the first lay member of the Florida Medical Association's Council on Ethical and Judicial Affairs, has served as lay representative on the Hillsborough County Medical Association's

Grievance Committee, serves on the board of St. Joseph's Hospital in Tampa, Florida, is on the National Board of the Tourette Syndrome Association, and was the community representative to the University of South Florida Medical School Self-Study Committee.

Note: From time to time throughout this book you'll find a pointer icon . This icon serves as a reminder that the information following it is important to remember.

CHAPTER 1

How Hospitals Differ

In a perfect world, there would be no disease, no disabilities, no disasters. No one would ever have any need to go to a hospital. Doctors, if they even existed in this fantasy world, would either pat us on the head to say how healthy we were or give us an apple each day to keep illness away.

Unfortunately, in real life, hospitals are a necessity, although their form and function have altered somewhat in the last decade and promise to change even more in the future. In a move by government and managed care organizations to cut costs, many services once performed within a hospital setting have been outsourced to what is referred to as "alternate site specialty care." These services may include, but are not limited to, rehabilitation, ambulatory surgery, infusion therapy, kidney dialysis, and subacute centers for patients whose conditions have stabilized but who require specialized treatment and continued medical supervision. While often offering the convenience of closer proximity to the patient's home and promising to improve the quality of care, the selection of what may be the "right" alternate site merely adds to the patient's confusion.

The decision of how to select a hospital and what type to choose often is surrendered to the physician in the hope that "he or she will know what's best for me." The fact that many doctors may have a financial interest in these institutions may be vaguely understood by patients and their families, but seldom are the implications of that marriage fully registered.

The selection of any type of health-care facility should not be made carelessly. The quality of the patient's care and the outcome of even a seemingly minor medical procedure may depend upon that choice. Your life or that of a loved one may hang in the balance of that decision. Yet most of us are far more diligent in gathering information before purchasing a new car, home, or television set than we are in determining to what health-care facility we'll entrust our life or that of someone important to us.

Choosing a hospital is a lot like selecting a potential spouse: You need to be aware of your priorities, check reputations, and get to know each other a little before saying "yes." Planning ahead in your hospital selection, before you actually need one, not only offers you a higher comfort level if you need to be admitted, but it also helps to prevent what could be a serious mismatch, a mistake that can't be turned around by anything as simple as a divorce.

TYPES OF HOSPITALS

Like spouses, hospitals come in many varieties. Your particular needs—both physical and emotional—as well as your pocketbook are important considerations. For the most part, level of care or services offered are the main bases for categorizing.

General Hospitals

A general hospital is one in which all or almost all medical services can be provided. These hospitals vary greatly in size. While the majority have fewer than 200 beds, many have more than 500 beds. While smaller hospitals may not enjoy the wealth of high-tech equipment as seems standard in the larger facilities today, communication may flow better in the smaller hospitals and the nursing staff may be more likely to remember you by name than "the bowel obstruction in room 603."

Most general hospitals offer care to everyone and treat nearly any type of medical condition. There are, however, general hospitals with no emergency department, no pediatrics department, and no facilities for obstetrics. In addition, nonprofit general hospitals with certain religious affiliations may not permit specific procedures, such as tubal ligations and therapeutic abortions, to be performed.

The majority of hospitals are allopathic, which means they are primarily staffed by medical doctors rather than by doctors of osteopathy, although in most areas of the United States D.O.s may enjoy staff privileges at these hospitals. There also are osteopathic hospitals, which differ little other than that they are staffed mainly by doctors of osteopathy. According to Eileen L. DiGiovanna, D.O., F.A.A.O., Assistant Dean of the New York College of Osteopathic Medicine, "The educational process is similar in both kinds of institutions. . . . The four years in osteopathic medical school are spent in the study of basic and clinical sciences, much as in allopathic medical schools, with added focus on osteopathic concepts and manipulation."[1]

Often, general acute-care hospitals have one or more departments that are more outstanding than others. Many times it's because a particular physician or group of physicians has an interest in that field and has built up that department. Never make a determination on which hospital to use based on a department's reputation alone, however. The doctor who "made" that department may be long gone, along with the expertise for which that department was noted.

Specialty Hospitals

Specialty hospitals are those caring for a particular type of patient—such as pediatrics or women—or those caring for patients with a particular medical need—such as bone disorders

---

[1]*Eileen L. DiGiovanna, D.O., F.A.A.O.,* Introduction to Osteopathic Medicine: An Osteopathic Approach to Diagnosis and Treatment, *ed. Eileen L. DiGiovanna, D.O., F.A.A.O. and Stanley Schiowitz, D.O., F.A.A.O. (Philadelphia: J.B. Lippincott Company, 1992), 1.*

(orthopedics); cancer (oncology); disorders of the ear, nose, or throat (otolaryngology); rehabilitation; or psychiatric problems.

Within this category are hospitals such as Shriners Hospitals for Children, a network of twenty-two pediatric hospitals (twenty in the United States, one in Mexico City, and one in Montreal), dedicated to serving children who have orthopedic problems, serious burn injuries, or spinal cord injuries. The families of these patients do not pay for their children's medical care, nor is there any third-party payment.

Teaching Hospitals

Most of us are familiar with the concept of teaching hospitals because television and the movies frequently use them as settings for dramatic (as well as comical) situations. The teaching hospital usually is affiliated with a medical school, which means patients are seen by medical students (who are not, as yet, "real" doctors), and by interns and residents (who are).

The good news about a teaching hospital is that generally it has state-of-the-art equipment and, because of its emphasis on research, may offer innovative treatment procedures, many of which have not, as yet, been written up in the journals. Teaching hospitals also tend to attract top specialists who are involved in research along with their teaching and patient-care duties.

The bad news about a teaching hospital is that medical students, interns, and residents are anxious to use this high-tech state-of-the-art equipment so sometimes patients have more tests (invasive and otherwise) than may be necessary. In addition, some of the treatment procedures, though innovative, may not prove effective over the long term.

Nonteaching Hospitals

A nonteaching hospital is staffed by licensed physicians who must apply for and receive "privileges" at that particular institution. (The staff also includes nursing staff, technicians, and others to be described later.) The attending physician may invite consultations by other physicians, but most of the time, the patient's care is in the hands of the attending physician and the nursing staff, which consists of registered nurses, licensed practical nurses, aides, and technical staff. If an emergency develops in a nonteaching facility, the nursing staff must contact your physician, who may be on the seventh tee with his or her portable phone turned off. You may have to settle for the covering physician.

Some people prefer the smaller community nonteaching hospital because they don't feel so overwhelmed. "I like the personal treatment," one patient told us. "It's like a neighborhood hospital. I'm not just a number. Besides, I'm only here for minor surgery." Her mistake was not realizing that there is no such thing as minor surgery. The doctor performing her "minor" surgery (removing three small rectal polyps) accidentally perforated her bowel. There was massive bleeding and she went into cardiac arrest. Her charming little hospital was not equipped to handle this type of dual emergency and she almost died.

This is not to say that all small community hospitals can't handle the unexpected. Many of them can and do and are excellent teaching institutions as well. The point is, you need to know what your intended hospital can do for you medically before you need its services.

HOW TO CHOOSE A HOSPITAL

Which type of hospital should you choose? Physicians themselves don't agree on which is better for the patient—the teaching or the nonteaching facility. Their preference is usually determined by their personal practice. While on the one hand the patient in a teaching hospital is assured of having a doctor available twenty-four hours a day, it's possible that the doctor may have just graduated from medical school three months ago and have little hands-on experience in dealing with a particular illness or emergency. He or she may attempt procedures (on you) that previously have only been observed, according to the "See one, do one, teach one," philosophy of some teaching hospitals.

Patients in a teaching hospital also must understand and accept that they may be the lesson-of-the-day, which means that students, interns, residents, and others being trained may examine and re-examine the subject, order invasive and expensive tests, and discuss the case in front of patients as though they were lab rats. If you're modest or if privacy is important to you, think twice about being admitted to a teaching hospital.

But, on the other hand, if an emergency arises in the middle of the night (and they often seem to), it's comforting to see an intern or resident who at least appears to know how to handle a crisis—and most of them do.

Teaching hospitals at medical centers generally are on the cutting edge of progressive experimental treatments that may become standard procedure once the information trickles down to other physicians throughout the land by way of journals, conventions, seminars, and workshops. While some doctors do use their computer modems to go on-line to gather the most up-to-date information on a particular disease or treatment procedure, the majority either don't have one or don't take the time to do so, or haven't ventured into wonderful Web world as yet.

Your Insurance Plan or Physician Choice May Dictate Your Choice of Hospital

Your choice of a hospital may be narrowed by your insurance plan or the physician you have already selected. Doctors must apply for staff privileges at hospitals to which they want to admit their patients. In smaller communities, there may be only one or two hospitals, so doctors may have privileges at one or both. But in cities with numerous hospitals, physicians must be selective, so they don't have to run all over town to make rounds. You may live near a particular hospital and want to be admitted there for the convenience of your family, only to find that your doctor does not have privileges there. While some hospitals may permit doctors to admit a few patients as a courtesy, most require physicians to apply for privileges (and guarantee that most of their patients will be admitted to that particular facility).

You also may find that your insurance plan lists specific hospitals where you must be admitted. While you still may choose to go to a different hospital if you so desire, your insurance may not cover as much (or any) of your expenses.

Whichever hospital you select, be sure that it has been accredited by the Joint Commission on Accreditation of Healthcare Organizations. This group, known as JCAHO, is an independent organization that makes regular inspections of health-care facilities and certifies that an institution's services and procedures are up to predetermined high standards. Although hospitals are not required to be inspected by JCAHO, most reputable institutions (80 percent of the nation's hospitals) do volunteer to be examined and accredited.

While some advocacy groups complain that JCAHO is too easy on hospitals, accrediting 99 percent of those surveyed, JCAHO's president, Dr. Dennis O'Leary, claims the system works. "Our public record speaks for itself. The Federal government has relied on our reports for over thirty years. So have Wall Street, education programs, and state agencies. We have the highest citation rate of any surveying organization. Our purpose is to get hospitals to fix their deficiencies and to improve their patient care, not to punish them. A hospital cited for deficiencies has three to six months to correct any problems our survey uncovers. Overall, we do find problems of one kind or another in 75 percent of the hospitals we inspect. Most of the hospitals value their accreditation; they fix their problems immediately."

To check on the accreditation of any hospital you're considering, contact the hospital or call the Joint Commission on Accreditation of Healthcare Organizations at (630) 792-5600. Their reports on individual hospital performances in fifty different areas are available to the public.

You also can check the American Hospital Association's (AHA's) *Guide to the Health Care Field* at your local library. Published annually, this directory lists all U.S. hospitals, noting those accredited by JCAHO. It also includes the type of hospital, number of beds, services, and other valuable information.

LOCATION, LOCATION, LOCATION

How important is location in your choice of a hospital? It could be extremely important, especially if you have a heart attack or a stroke. Time is of the essence and an extra fifteen minutes getting to the hospital of your choice could mean the difference between life and death. That's why emergency medical services (EMS) in many communities are expected to bring a patient to the closest hospital, unless the patient (or family member) disagrees. You can always be transferred to your preferred hospital after your condition is stabilized.

Your personal safety at the hospital is another consideration in making your selection, one so important that we have devoted an entire chapter (Chapter 5) to this issue. In many communities, hospitals, especially their emergency departments, have become war zones. Stress, gangs, drugs, and fear make emotions highly charged. In addition, many general hospitals are located in transitional areas in order to be easily accessible to the general population or public transportation. Unfortunately, this is often the area with the highest crime rates as well.

Take this issue seriously when making your selection of a hospital. Check out the hospital at night to see if the parking areas are lighted and patrolled by security staff.

SEE FOR YOURSELF

If at all possible, eyeball the entire hospital yourself, rather than relying on its public relations materials to tell you about the physical plant. Pictures *do* lie, as many college students have discovered to their dismay when they arrive on campus and see their dorm room for the first time.

Although you can contact the public relations department and ask for a tour of the hospital, remember that they probably use their brightest and most verbal volunteers for that task, reminding them to stay away from areas that need refurbishing or repairing. You'll probably learn more by just dropping in for lunch at the cafeteria and eavesdropping on staff and visitors' conversations or by visiting a friend who's a patient there. We know of one enterprising man who was scouting out hospitals for his wife's elective surgery. He bought a floral arrangement at the hospital's gift shop and just picked a room at random to deliver it.

"I learned a lot," he said. "Too much to make me want to be admitted to that particular hospital. Soiled linen was piled up in a bin outside one of the patient's rooms. There were half-eaten food trays left over from lunch two hours earlier stacked nearby on a cart, and after looking at the mess, I could only marvel that even half of the meal had been eaten. The nurses were gossiping, disregarding patients' call bells. The waiting room area was filled with crumpled newspapers and dirty coffee cups, and the halls smelled of urine. I'm glad I took the time to see the place firsthand," he said. "Their brochure had made the place almost look like a spa or resort hotel. But after what I saw, I shuddered to think what quality of care my wife might have received there."

Cleanliness in a hospital has far more than just aesthetic value. Open wounds, compromised immune systems, and lowered resistance make patients extremely vulnerable to the dangers of infection. According to the Hospital Infections Program of the Federal Centers for Disease Control and Prevention, each year about two million Americans develop nosocomial infections (hospital-acquired infections). These infections have the potential to invade tissues and become extremely serious. Sometimes they even may be fatal.

Before selecting a hospital, contact its risk management department (not the public relations department). Ask about their nosocomial infection rate and whether they have a designated infection control staff member; its nurse/patient ratio and if these are registered nurses (RNs) or licensed practical nurses (LPNs); and its rate of medication errors and what procedures are in place to prevent these mistakes from occurring. If they refuse to give you this information, find another hospital if at all possible. Although hospitals are not obligated to give out this information, they should welcome patients who understand the importance of these statistics. Informed patients help hospitals to reduce human errors.

CHAPTER 2

Getting to Know the Area

There are two ways to get into the hospital as a patient—through the emergency room and through the admitting office. According to Dr. Arthur L. Kellermann of Emory University Schools of Medicine and Public Health, "Nationwide, approximately 40 percent of hospital inpatients are admitted through the emergency department." Both avenues of entry can cause unbelievable delays and anxiety, yet you can (and should) preplan for either entrance.

THE EMERGENCY DEPARTMENT

Recent television shows have spotlighted and glamorized hospital emergency departments. While it's true that real-life drama takes place in this area of the hospital, TV viewers may have unrealistic expectations and be surprised and dismayed when they experience firsthand that the health-care professionals in many ER departments are too overworked and understaffed to be able to spend "quality time" with their patients.

What Is an "Emergency Room?"

What constitutes the emergency room varies from one hospital to another. Other than in the smallest of rural hospitals, it's actually a department and not merely a room. In one institution, the emergency department may be primarily a treatment center, where critical cases are given supportive care before they are admitted to the hospital. In another, the emergency room may be like a mini-hospital, with casting rooms for broken bones, operating rooms for minor surgeries, and X ray and other diagnostic facilities. Some larger general hospitals may have separate pediatric emergency departments while many hospitals may have no emergency room facilities at all.

In the 1980s, realizing that serious accident victims receiving appropriate trauma care within the first hour had the best chance of survival, the American College of Surgeons' Committee on Trauma set standards for emergency trauma care. Their designation of a Level I trauma center is the highest ranking. It means that a designated trauma team is always within the hospital and ready to respond instantaneously. Trauma team members, all specialists in trauma treatment, have the training and experience to rapidly diagnose severe problems and to immediately take appropriate action.

Level I also means that a trauma treatment room equipped with state-of-the-art equipment is always available for seriously injured patients and that a trauma operating room is always ready for surgery.

A Level II trauma center is at a slightly lesser state of readiness in that the designated trauma center staff may not necessarily be in the hospital, but must be available within thirty minutes after a trauma alert is called.[1]

Obviously, you can't predict where you might be in case of a serious accident, but it's important to know whether there's a Level I or Level II trauma center in your community and if so, at which hospital. Call the nonemergency telephone number of your local fire/rescue department or the larger hospitals in your area for this information. Also check to see if your insurance covers you at that facility.

---

[1] *Adapted from an article written by Sandra Zec in Tampa General Hospital's magazine,* In General, *Issue 6, Spring 1966.*

How Are Emergency Rooms Staffed?

The staffing of emergency rooms depends on the type of hospital. A teaching hospital's emergency room is largely staffed by interns and residents, graduates of medical school who are in rotation— that is, spending a set period of time training in the ER before moving on to experience pediatrics, obstetrics, or some other medical specialty. Emergency rooms also may be staffed by:

- Private practice physicians who alternate being on call for ER service

- Medical personnel hired by companies that contract to run emergency rooms

- Moonlighting residents in other specialities

- One or more of the approximately 12,786 board-certified emergency room physicians. This medical specialty is a fairly new one, officially recognized as such in 1980. The American Board of Emergency Medicine certifies the competence of physicians who are specially trained in this field.

Registered nurses, licensed practical nurses, respiratory therapists, clerks, and technicians round out most ER staffs. The nursing and technical staff usually remains constant with only the physicians' roster rotating.

With this variety of possibilities, the quality of care varies greatly from one emergency department to another. According to Jim Keaney, M.D., M.P.H., and author of *The Rape of Emergency Medicine,* many hospitals—especially those with commercially contracted emergency department staffs—may have poorly trained, nonboard-certified physicians staffing their emergency departments. According to the American Board of Emergency Medicine, fewer than half of the 25,000 doctors working in U.S. emergency departments are board-certified emergency physicians. A study by the Josiah Macy, Jr., Foundation revealed that only 19 percent of our nation's 111 Veterans Affairs hospitals employ emergency physicians who are residency trained, board certified, or both.[2] Less experienced than a board-certified emergency room physician, many of these "fill-in" doctors have made serious, even fatal errors. A former emergency department nurse told peers she retired rather than work with nonboard-certified ER physicians who resorted to using "cheat sheets to check on how to perform certain procedures."

Of course, board-certified physicians have been known to make serious mistakes as well, but the ER physician who is board certified should have acquired the broad spectrum of skills needed for this high-pressured specialty.

In 1988, an ER physician not certified in emergency medicine attempted to intubate his patient, an eighteen-year-old slightly injured in a car accident. The doctor inserted a breathing tube into the boy's esophagus, instead of his trachea. Rather than providing oxygen to the young man's lungs, which would continue the flow of oxygenated blood to the boy's brain, the oxygen filled his stomach. Within the hour, the boy was brain dead.

Emergency medicine is a challenging specialty. The staff never knows who the next patient will be or what problems he or she will bring in. It could be anything from a drug overdose to an impending birth with placenta previa, a massive gun shot wound to a poisonous snake bite. According to Dr. Larry Bedard, president of the American College of Emergency Physicians and member of President Clinton's Task Force on Violence Against Women, "About 20 percent of women treated in emergency departments are there for injuries or illnesses associated with domestic violence." The response for this variety of emergencies must be immediate and skillful. The emergency department is no place for a hospital to try to cut corners to save money. Besides evaluating and treating an average of twenty-five to forty patients during an

---

[2] Josiah Macy, Jr., Foundation, "The Role of Emergency Medicine in the Future of American Medical Care," Annals of Emergency Medicine 25 (1995): 230–233.

eight- to twelve-hour shift, emergency physicians handle thirty-five to forty telephone calls, supervise nonphysician Emergency Department (ED) staff, interact with emergency medical service (EMS) personnel and law enforcement officers, and talk with family members or others who accompany the patient to the emergency department.[3]

Often a nurse acts as an intake or "triage" person to determine which patient is the greatest emergency, although some states now require that only physicians serve this function. Emergency departments are not like bakeries where you take a number and first come is first served. Instead, the most serious cases receive top priority. If you've come for a slightly sprained ankle, be prepared to wait, sometimes for hours.

On the other hand, if it's chest pains or something that is potentially serious, this is the time to be assertive. An infected spider bite may be painful and require treatment; however, a bite from a recluse spider or fire ant, especially to someone highly allergic to the venom, along with other hypersensitives can cause anaphylactic shock in a matter of minutes, which could be fatal. Don't be reticent; speak up.

The American College of Emergency Physicians urges you to learn the following warning signs of a medical emergency:

- Difficulty in breathing or shortness of breath

- Chest or upper abdominal pain or pressure

- Fainting

- Sudden dizziness

- Weakness or change in vision

- Confusion in mental status

- Any sudden, severe pain

[3] G. C. Hamilton, *"Introduction to Emergency Medicine,"* in G. C. Hamilton, A. B. Sanders, G. R. Strange, A. T. Trott, eds., Emergency Medicine: An Approach to Clinical Problem Solving *(Philadelphia: W. B. Saunders, 1991), 3–18.*

- Bleeding that won't stop
- Severe or persistent vomiting
- Coughing up blood or vomiting blood
- Suicidal or homicidal feelings

☞ Always tell the triage person if you've had bad reactions to a particular substance before, your throat is closing up, you feel uneasy, there's a ringing in your ears, or you're having trouble breathing. These symptoms can develop in a matter of minutes, so don't be polite and wait your turn and don't be put off by a staff person who minimizes your symptoms.

Unfortunately, most ERs are overcrowded with people who really do not have a medical emergency. It's estimated that fewer than 60 percent of those seeking treatment in an emergency room really need to be there. The remaining 40+ percent either have conditions that could have waited until their doctor's office or clinic opened the next day, didn't want to bother their own physician, or don't have a doctor and use the ER as their personal walk-in clinic. Yet, according to Dr. Robert Shesser of George Washington University School of Medicine, "Emergency departments serve as a much needed safety net for those who have no other source of medical care, as well as for thousands of other Americans when they are traveling."

How Should You Select an Emergency Room?

Often you don't have the luxury to choose where you go or are taken. Either there's been an accident or sudden illness and the ambulance takes you to the closest emergency facility or you're visiting an area, have a medical emergency, and just head to the nearest hospital. If you do have a choice, however, follow these guidelines:

- Don't use an emergency room as your primary physician. You'll pay far more (some studies say double) and probably wait longer in an ER for a nonemergency condition.

- Check out your local emergency rooms before you need one. See if they're clean, have seating for all their patients and families, and have easy access to water fountains, rest rooms, and telephones. You may be spending hours there.

- The cleanliness aspect is more than just an aesthetic one. There are many drug-resistant diseases such as certain types of pneumonia and tuberculosis, as well as colds, flu, eye infections, and so on that can be spread by using dirty towels, touching surfaces and then putting your fingers in your mouth or nose or rubbing your eyes. If the waiting room and rest rooms look dirty, they probably are breeding grounds for bacteria.

- A few hospital emergency rooms, such as the one in Bergan Mercy Medical Center in Omaha, have gone out of their way to reduce the anxiety levels of visitors to their departments. Among other changes, they moved crash carts, wheelchairs, and other stress-inducing equipment to out-of-sight storage areas. They also added rocking chairs to pediatric exam rooms, along with VCRs, so children can be distracted by cartoons while being stitched up or examined.

- Be sure there are security guards conspicuously present. Many victims of violence arrive at the ER with concealed weapons. Reduce your chances of being injured or even killed in a crossfire.

- Ask if the hospital provides escorts to accompany you to the parking lots at night. When you're anxious about a loved one or have just received emergency medical treatment yourself, your guard may be down—a sure way to attract attention from someone loitering near the hospital looking for a pigeon to rob.

- If you're pregnant, have children, or have a chronic medical condition, be sure the hospital has the proper facilities to treat you or other members of your family if you should need to be admitted. "People can be unreasonable," said one emergency room physician. "They bring their kids here because we're nearby and then get angry when we can't admit their youngsters because this hospital doesn't have a pediatric unit."

If you do have children, it is extremely important to check out emergency rooms at your local hospitals. In one year in the United States, injury alone is likely to take the lives of more than 20,000 children under the age of nineteen. Ask if there are pediatric specialists on staff, including a pediatric anesthesiologist.

According to Donald N. Medearis, Jr., M.D., Charles Wilder Professor of Pediatrics at Harvard Medical School and chief of Children's Services at Massachusetts General Hospital in Boston, "It is vital to have experienced pediatric health-care practitioners caring for children in the emergency department. Children are not merely 'little adults.' They are smaller and proportioned differently. A child's normal respiratory rate, heart rate, and blood pressure are all different from an adult's. Characteristic changes in those vital signs that signal deterioration in adults may not be present in children. Stages in children's physiologic, emotional, and behavioral development affect their responses to medical care.

"For these and other reasons, different and special equipment and expertise must be in place to care for children in emergency situations. There must be different-sized instruments, different doses, and different kinds of medications, and different ways to give the psychological support that a dangerously ill or severely injured child might need."[4]

- Determine the qualifications of the staff at the particular ER facility you're considering. If you have a chronic condition such as heart disease or asthma, be comfortable that the staff is trained to treat your type of emergencies.

- If you or a family member has difficulty speaking or understanding English, ask if a *professional* medical interpreter is on staff. While many physicians and nurses may think they are fluent in another language, such as Spanish or French, studies show that their proficiency is limited when explaining medical issues.

- Be certain the specific hospital you select is on your insurance plan before you need to go there. Many people don't know the rules of their HMO or PPO or show up at the wrong hospital. Many health plans want to keep their subscribers out of the emergency room whenever possible. You may be fully liable for the bill.

There also is a growing trend for insurers to pay for emergency treatment based on a patient's diagnosis, instead of his or her symptoms. This presents a real dilemma, according to Dr. Gregory Henry, president of the American College of Emergency Physicians. "Today, emergency physicians can literally stop a heart attack in progress if the patient gets to the emergency room in time, and we may soon be able to do the same thing for stroke. You can see patients [coming into the ER] seeking treatment for symptoms that can

[4]*Taken from a speech by Donald N. Medearis, Jr., M.D., Charles Wilder Professor of Pediatrics, Harvard Medical School, and chief of children's services at Massachusetts General Hospital in Boston, delivered in Washington, D.C., July 7, 1993.*

indeed be life-threatening, even though their final diagnosis may be for a more minor condition. The patient who comes in with chest pain, but leaves with 'general symptoms' may be out of luck when it comes to getting the bill paid."

- Find out whether there are ER isolation rooms for people with multidrug-resistant tuberculosis or other highly contagious conditions. Most hospitals keep these patients waiting in the emergency room until an isolation bed opens within the hospital. You and your family can be exposed to these serious medical problems as you wait for your turn to see a physician.

Appearing on the "Donahue" television show, Jim Keaney, M.D., M.P.H., and author of *The Rape of Emergency Medicine*, offered these suggestions for preselecting emergency medical facilities: "Before you need an emergency department, call the hospital to ask about their ER team. Is it locally based or are the physicians flown in from somewhere else? Is the emergency department contracted out to a commercial company or is it part of the hospital's facilities? How long have the physicians been there?" We offer one additional question: Are the physicians staffing the emergency department trained and certified in emergency medicine?

These physicians can mean the difference between life and death for you or your loved ones. Often, in a true emergency, you may have no say where you are taken; if you do have a choice, doing your homework in advance can make a difference.

How to Help the Emergency Room Personnel Help You

According to emergency-room physicians, patients and their families can play an important part in improving the care and eventual outcome when coming for treatment in the emergency room. They offer these guidelines:

- Carry a card in your wallet listing and identifying all medications you are taking. This is especially important if you are a caregiver for an elderly parent. It is not uncommon for people in their seventies and eighties to be taking ten or more medications each day. It's vital for the emergency-room staff to be aware of what these drugs are so they don't use anything that will adversely interact with the present drugs in the patient's system.

  This information could have saved the life of Libby Zion, daughter of New York journalist Sidney Zion. She died after being given Demerol, which should not be taken with Nardil, a medication that she was taking for depression.

- Use that same card to inform the emergency-room staff of any allergies you have in connection to a particular medication. Don't wait for them to ask; give them the card with that information. Serious drug allergies can quickly trigger cardiac arrest or anaphylactic shock.

- Also use that card to describe your past medical history. If they don't know you have an ulcer, for example, they may give you Motrin or another anti-inflammatory drug that could cause internal bleeding. The drug Coumadin should be used with special precaution on patients taking Dilantin for seizures. Even something as common as aspirin, which you may be taking for a heart problem or an arthritic condition, may interact dangerously with other medications. As there are far too many possibly dangerous drug interactions to list here, protect yourself by always listing every medication you're taking, including vitamins and other over-the-counter preparations.

- Verify all information before signing any forms. Be sure that the clerk has typed in the proper name, age, and medical data. Names such as "Johnson" and "Johnston" appear similar, but such an error can be deadly when it comes to confusion during treatment. In some ER facilities, clerks type in the patient's allergies. Check to be sure that all of yours have been properly identified. Be certain that the site of your problem has been correctly recorded, such as "left eye" or "right hip."

- Give your most serious complaint first. Don't say, "Oh, I'm tired all the time," if you've come in because of chest pain or complain of a nosebleed if you've had nasal hemorrhaging for an hour. If your child's accidentally been poisoned, bring the container or plant with you.

- Tell the truth. If you smoke or use illegal drugs, don't hide it from the emergency-room staff. They won't be judgmental. According to a study published in the December 1995 issue of *Annuals of Emergency Medicine*, nearly half of all emergency-department patients aged thirty-one to forty complaining of chest pain had recently used cocaine. Dr. Judd E. Hollander, lead author of the study and an emergency physician, stressed that if patients who have recently used cocaine are treated with the same methods as patients who have not used cocaine, they could experience life-threatening complications. Cocaine toxins can severely affect the coronary arteries, so it's important to report cocaine and other illegal drug use. Lying about it could kill you.

- If you use herbal therapies such as ginseng, licorice, and lycium, be sure to tell the emergency-room physician about it. Many herbal mixtures are adulterated with common pain relievers that can cause bleeding ulcers.

- If you have an advanced directive—a legal document describing your choices concerning medical care—or if you are a caregiver for someone who does, bring it with you.

- Know the date of your last tetanus shot. Guidelines suggest booster shots every ten years. If you have a puncture wound and don't remember when you last had a tetanus immunization, you'll probably get another. In the United States, 59 percent of the cases of tetanus and 75 percent of the deaths occur in persons sixty years of age or older.[5] Therefore, many hospitals routinely administer tetanus toxoid injections to all adult patients unless the person's physician orders it not to be given.

- If the patient is a child, an elderly person, someone who doesn't speak English, or otherwise has difficulty communicating, insist on staying with him or her in the treatment area to translate or help decipher responses. It's frightening enough to be in an emergency room. Imagine the terror of knowing you have no way to communicate where and how you hurt.

Although you may spend hours in the waiting room of an emergency department, you can help to influence the quality of the medical care you or a loved one gets in this facility. Do your homework; know your rights; protect your well-being.

[5]*Centers for Disease Control, "Surveillance of Tetanus—United States, 1989–1990,"* MMWR Morb Mortal Weekly Report SS-8, 41 (1992): 1–9.

ADMITTING OFFICE

The second way to enter a hospital is through the admitting office. Patients entering by this route have nonemergency conditions and are expected by the staff. You should have been given pre-admissions forms by the physician admitting you to the hospital. Take time to complete these forms carefully. Print or type your responses. Answer all the questions and do so honestly. Your use of alcohol or illegal drugs can alter the effects of medications and anesthetics you may be given. Asking for your medical history is more than an idle curiosity. The information can alert the staff to problems that may arise.

If the patient is your child or teenager, take advantage of the many books available in bookstores and the library that describe the hospital routines and environment. If the hospital offers a pre-admissions tour, take it. Becoming familiar with the surroundings may help a child feel less anxious. If your youngster is old enough to ask questions of the doctors, nurses, and technicians, encourage him or her to be assertive.

Most patients are given an exact time to present themselves to the admitting office at a hospital. The majority of them arrive precisely on time with their little overnight bag by their side, then wonder why they must wait for an hour or so before being admitted. When we asked hospital administrators why this occurred, they either sidestepped the question or explained, "Well, it's hard to know how long each admissions takes. . . ."

Don't sit silently letting the cobwebs grow as your blood pressure soars. After twenty minutes or so of waiting, find someone who seems to be in authority and remind him or her of your presence. Files, charts, and sign-in sheets do get lost. Your name may have been checked off by mistake, without your being called into one of the cubicles usually found in admissions departments. If you're still ignored, ask to see the hospital administrator. Your active participation within the hospital begins here.

When you do get in to see the admitting person, answer all questions truthfully. Insist on privacy during the admitting procedure. You don't need to answer personal questions with a room full of strangers eavesdropping. If you don't understand the questions or need an interpreter, request help. If you have an allergy to any type of medication, be sure it is marked on your admitting forms as well as the identification bracelet you're given.

While some hospitals wait until you're actually in your assigned room and checked in by the nursing staff to give you an allergy bracelet, don't assume this to be so. Ask when you will receive your allergy bracelet. It could save your life.

Private Room versus Semi-Private

As with so many things in life, there is no one "right" answer to the question of whether a private or semi-private room is preferable. For the most part, however, we feel you're safer paying extra for a private room if you possibly can afford it. The only advantages we see to a semi-private room are:

- You have someone to talk to if you really feel up to it.

- If you need a nurse in a hurry, there's someone else to call for help—providing, of course, the roommate is conscious, comprehends what you're saying, and is able to speak.

- If you fall out of bed or trip on the way to the bathroom, your roommate can ring for help—providing, of course, that the roommate notices, is conscious, and realizes that something is wrong.

The disadvantages of a semi-private room are many:

- If your roommate has an infection, such as staph, you may catch it.

- If your roommate's visitors have infections, you are exposed to them as well.

- Your physicians may carry infection to you by not washing their hands after touching the door handle and then coming to check you. The handle could easily become contaminated by bacteria after your roommate's physicians or nurses change a dressing, empty a bedpan, or touch a surface and then touch the door handle without washing their hands. Bacteria and viruses can live a long time on a surface, just waiting to be picked up and moved on to another source—you.

- Your rest may be disturbed by your roommate's moaning, phone calls, visitors, or television viewing habits, and by the nursing staff or technicians popping in and out of the room.

- Shared bathroom facilities between roommates can encourage the exchange of bacteria on surfaces.

- Elderly patients may become confused with the added commotion of visitors and medical personnel visiting their roommate.

- Food trays may be mixed between beds in semi-private rooms, with one patient receiving food that is contraindicated either because of a certain type of medicine being taken or because of a specific disorder—such as pie or cake for someone with diabetes, a cheese dish for someone taking a specific type of antidepressant, or a high-sodium meal for someone with high blood pressure.

- You may wind up getting medication or treatment procedures prescribed for your roommate by mistake. Just as a Jewish woman received last rites from the priest who mistook her for her Catholic roommate, a tired resident or nurse may get mixed up and hang the wrong medication on your IV stand.

- Children of all ages should have a private room.

Although some pediatric facilities formerly encouraged semi-private rooms or four-bed wards for their young patients, the trend since the 1970s has been for private rooms with sleeping-in facilities for a parent.

Insist on your right to stay with your sick child. According to the American Academy of Pediatrics, "Many sick children benefit emotionally and physically from having their parents participate in their hospital care . . . parent participation also might reduce the cost of hospital care of the sick child."[6]

Even more important, you need to stay with your infant or young child to ask important questions when necessary and to learn exactly which medications and treatments are being given to your youngster, why, and what side effects they may have. It also assures that you are in the room with your child when the physician or consultant comes by.

While adolescents, struggling for a sense of independence, may consider themselves "too grown-up" to have a parent staying with them, they still need you nearby to act as their advocate. If your teenager is in a semi-private room, insist that the hospital provides you with a private area so you can meet with your youngster to discuss possible treatments, listen to questions and fears, talk over possible side effects of medications, and so on. Many hospitals have rooms set aside for parents of older children that serve to give the

[6]*Committee on Hospital Care, American Academy of Pediatrics, Joseph M. Garfunkel, M.D., and Hugh E. Evans, M.D., eds.,* Hospital Care of Children and Youth, *(Elk Grove Village, IL: American Academy of Pediatrics, 1986): 119.*

youngsters their "space," yet offer the security of having Mom or Dad nearby to ask or answer questions and to give emotional support.

LABORATORIES

Although you may never see the inside of a hospital laboratory because usually the laboratory technicians come to the patient's bedside, you still need to be aware of this area of the hospital. Your life may depend it.

Many of your treatment procedures and actual diagnosis may be based solely on the outcome of the tests analyzed in the laboratory. Too often, however, the results are erroneous, giving the physician relying on them either false negatives or false positives. You, in turn, may then be subject to painful procedures including, but not limited to, surgery and improper medications. You actually could die because a lab technician was overtired and mislabeled or misread your slide, performed a test improperly, or was otherwise careless. Recently, cases of women whose pap tests were misdiagnosed as normal when they actually contained cancer cells were made public. Some of these women died from their disease, which, if diagnosed earlier, might have been cured.

The seemingly simple act of typing the report or entering codes relating to laboratory data can also lead to dangerous assumptions. A young woman, being followed up for breast cancer, was amazed to see "multiple myeloma" typed in on the diagnosis section of the papers sent to her insurance company. She scurried back to her oncologist in alarm. He assured her that there was no sign of multiple myeloma, an often fatal disease. The clerk had typed in the wrong code. It took months of letters and phone calls to get the misinformation out of her insurance company's computer (and she suspects that it is still drifting about somewhere in the hospital's never-never land of computer bits and bytes).

Additional factors that may lead to problems in laboratories include improper handling of the specimen so that it is contaminated, poor temperature control, actually losing the specimen altogether so that another test must be performed, mislabeling it, failing to secure an adequate amount for testing, delay in getting the specimen to the laboratory, and failing to conduct the testing under proper conditions, such as doing a stool sample without telling the patient to refrain from eating red meat and other foods that might alter the test results. Mistakes also are made by harried and fatigued lab technicians trying to read more tests in a day than they should. What's more, 25 percent of all lab tests that are done—correctly or incorrectly—are never even seen by the doctor. The report either does not make it to the patient's file or, if it does, the physician doesn't read it. Sloppy? Yes. Dangerous? It certainly could be.

Lab tests were never meant to replace a physician's personal observations and insights from carefully taking a patient's history. Yet many doctors rely too heavily on the results of tests, ignoring the fact that they may have been contaminated by some form of human error. Even more frightening, many HMOs deny payment for retesting, so the physicians who question lab results hesitate to order them a second time at the patient's expense.

X-RAY DEPARTMENT

The X-ray department seems to hold the greatest fear for many patients. It's usually located in the bowels of the hospital, and the patient is taken (often at night) down on a gurney or in a wheelchair and left to wait in the hall. Frequently there's a row of people waiting, some of whom are crying children and others, confused and frightened elderly people. Once inside, the patient is positioned, told not to move, and left alone on a cold and hard table under a massive machine.

Always accompany your family member down to the X-ray department. The waits are usually long and the technicians tend to forget they are working with a human being, not just a spine, chest, or neck. They also have been known to mix-up patients and

X-ray the wrong part of the anatomy, which causes that patient to have additional radiation (and discomfort, in some cases) if and when the error is discovered and corrected.

Many pediatric hospitals, like some of the units in the Shriners Hospitals system, understand how frightening the X-ray room can be when you are isolated with its huge impersonal equipment. They decorate their X-ray departments to be child-friendly by painting the walls with pictures of benevolent pirates and treasure chests, animals, and fish. The illustrations distract the children's attention so they remain motionless when the X ray is taken. This reduces the number of retakes required, thus exposing the children to less radiation.

The elderly may also become confused during an X ray. Ask the technician to explain the procedures in front of you. If you think your elderly family member doesn't understand, rephrase the explanation. Stay with your loved one until the technician is ready to take the picture. Then tell your family member that you have to go behind the lead screen, but that you will be right back as soon as the X ray has been taken. Most uncooperative elderly patients are frightened, not contrary.

INTENSIVE CARE UNITS

It's ironic that the areas devoted to those most ill are filled with the greatest amount of technology, little, if any, privacy, continual overhead lighting, and noise pollution, all creating an impersonal environment. In addition, caring loved ones are kept at a distance, except for carefully monitored visiting periods.

The ICU is expensive, far more than a normal hospital room, because of the intensity of the nursing care. It also is a breeding ground of germ sharing because of the severity of the illnesses of its patients. Elderly and pediatric patients can easily become frightened and confused by the constant noise, commotion, and lack of a sense of night and day, which slows their recovery and negates their cooperative spirit.

Despite the fact that there really is no physical space for you to squeeze yourself in next to your family member—and sitting on the bed is against the rules—make friends with the ICU staff and plead for every extra opportunity for a quick visit. If that cannot be arranged, keep the communication lines open at all times. Remember that most ICU staffs are overworked and do their job in the most stressful of conditions. Don't add to their tension; the mistake they make due to fatigue might be with your loved one.

Do be sympathetic to the staff. They're dealing with constant life-and-death situations with extremely ill patients. They'll appreciate your bringing in bagels, cookies, or other snacks to munch on to help lower their stress levels.

Don't bring flowers or other gifts to a loved one in the ICU, however. There's no place to put them and chances are the patient wouldn't notice or appreciate them anyway.

If you're the patient in the ICU, chances are you won't be able to look out for your own well-being. Try to have a family member or friend who will.

CHAPTER 3

The Hospital's Cast of Characters

B ecoming familiar with the players in the hospital drama is important for many reasons, all of which could save your life or that of a loved one.

First of all, knowing the cast of characters gives you an idea of the vast number of people involved with any patient's care, even in a relatively small hospital or when dealing with a so-called "minor" procedure. When you understand how many people are involved, you begin to see how easily mistakes can be made because of ignorance, miscommunication, sloppiness, and, all too commonly, human error.

THERE ARE NO MINOR PLAYERS

Just as the success of a theater production or movie depends on the talents and teamwork of the entire cast and crew, from lighting and sound technicians to makeup experts, wardrobe stylists, and dressers, it isn't only the stars who are important within the hospital. The minor roles are equally important in achieving and maintaining high-quality care, including those people you may never see, such as the laboratory technician who reads your slides or the pharmacist who fills your prescriptions. Even the transporter, who seemingly has nothing more important to do than to push your wheelchair or gurney to the X-ray department or therapy room, must be sure that he or she gets the right patient at the right time to the right place, and does so safely. Countless patients have found themselves having uncomfortable upper or lower G.I. barium X rays and other invasive tests, only to discover later that the procedure was intended for the patient in the other bed or from the room next door.

Once you know the job description and experience required of the personnel charged with your health care, you begin to gain an understanding and appreciation of what they know (or should know). This enables you to ask the charge nurse (who is usually a registered nurse) to come in to answer a question because you'll know that a registered nurse's training is far more extensive than that of an LPN (licensed practical nurse), a nurse's aide, or a patient care assistant.

☞ Take time to learn the names of those whose shifts are on the floor (or wing) of your room at the hospital. Calling someone by name helps to personalize you or your family member so you're not just "the hernia in bed two." It also protects you if you can tell the charge nurse, "Sheila gave me my Procardia an hour ago. She must have forgotten to chart it," rather than saying, "It was a pretty nurse with blond hair . . . or maybe it was the redhead."

You need to do everything you can (short of redecorating your room with flowered wallpaper and an antique rug) to insure that the nursing staff remembers who you are to prevent misidentifications from taking place. Put a family picture in an inexpensive frame (you'd be surprised what disappears in a hospital, so don't use your favorite sterling silver frame). It gives the medical staff a chance to make conversation, asking how old the kids are, the dog's name, and so on, while subtly reminding them that you are an individual with a life other than just that of a patient.

☞ Ask the nurse if there are others on your floor or wing of the hospital with your same (or similar) last name. There shouldn't be; if there are, ask to be transferred or have a warning bracelet added to the others you're now wearing. Harried nurses, technicians, and transporters are supposed to check wristbands before dispensing medicine to patients, drawing blood, taking a patient to another part of the hospital for treatment, or disconnecting a ventilator. But a quick glance might not discern the difference between Betty Weiss and Bette Weis or John Wentworth and John Wintworth. "What's in a name?" William Shakespeare asked. The answer is painfully obvious: At times, it may be the difference between life and death.

Ask a friend or family member to leave a box of cookies, fruit, or candy at the nursing station. This isn't a bribe, but rather a thank-you gesture in advance. While flowers are also nice, their care means extra work for the nurses and they don't need additional tasks that take time away from their patients.

DOCTORS

How to Select a Physician

Selecting a physician used to be strictly a personal choice. Someone needing a doctor would ask friends, business associates, the local medical association, or the nearby hospital for a list of names. When a few names kept appearing, a choice would be made from that group.

Today, with HMOs (health maintenance organizations), PPOs (preferred provider organizations), and other third-person providers, most individuals are assigned a list of physicians enrolled in that particular program. You must make a selection from that list. This makes it even more vital for you to carefully check out each doctor you are considering. Don't let close proximity be the only deciding factor. It may be far wiser driving fifteen minutes farther to get a physician with stronger credentials, who is board certified in his or her specialty, and with whom you can develop a trusting relationship.

But don't think of an M.D. (medical doctor) as being the only type of physician available. Six percent of all U.S. physicians are D.O.s (doctors of osteopathic medicine). According to John P. Sevastos, D.O., president of The American Osteopathic Association, "D.O.s have essentially the same qualifications, medical education, internship, licensure, and specialties as M.D.s. They are equal with M.D.s under the laws of all fifty states, serve as commissioned officers in the medical corps of all armed forces, plus the Veterans Administration and Public Health Service. And they are recognized as physicians by the A.M.A. Moreover, 31 percent of the profession is board certified in a full range of medical specialties, including surgery, anesthesiology, emergency medicine, psychiatry, obstetrics, pediatrics, radiology, and others."

While both receive similar training, medical doctors tend to specialize early on in their training, while D.O.s generally begin with family practice and then specialize. Central to osteopathic medicine is the body's musculoskeletal system (including bones, muscles, tendons, tissues, nerves and spinal column) and its importance to a patient's well-being. D.O.s view the human body as an integrated whole, with a fundamental concern with the entire body, preventive medicine, holistic medicine, proper diet, and keeping the patient fit, although these distinctions between D.O.s and M.D.s have blurred somewhat in recent years.

"Another difference," said Scott M. Chase, a doctor of osteopathic medicine in general practice in Maine, "is manipulation of the muscular/skeletal system and a laying on of hands, which is often part of the therapeutic treatment." Dr. Chase, like a growing number of D.O.s, is in a medical practice with both M.D.s and D.O.s. Most allopathic hospitals in the United States grant privileges to D.O.s as well as M.D.s.

The managed care restriction limiting free choice in selecting your physician makes your decision more difficult, and even more important, because it is vital—life saving in many cases—for you to select a physician who has had proper training, and is one with whom you can communicate and feel confidence. This doctor will often be the "gate keeper," the individual who holds the power to refer you to a specialist or to prevent your seeing one.

Capitation—an insurance situation in which your primary physician is given a specific amount of money for each patient, which is lessened each time a patient is sent to a specialist—may encourage some physicians to treat a case themselves, rather than referring the patient to a specialist. By the time these doctors realize that they may be over their heads and decide to send the patient to an expert who deals with complex cases, the disorder may have become more serious and more difficult to treat. Sometimes, as has happened with women suffering from ovarian cancer who finally are permitted to see a specialist, the disease is too advanced to be treated successfully.

So take your time in determining who will be your "gate keeper." Your life may depend upon it.

If you are over sixty-five, look for a doctor who specializes in geriatric medicine, if at all possible. It may be difficult as, according to the Alliance for Aging Research, there are only 7,000 of them in the United States. Less than 3 percent of medical school graduates have any training in geriatrics at all, despite the fact that by the middle of the next century, one in five Americans will be sixty-five or over. Yet as we get older, our body chemistry changes and medications are metabolized differently. Some conditions that may seem irreversible to a physician not familiar with geriatric medicine often can be treated successfully by someone who is.

With the growing number of women doctors (20 percent of doctors in the United States today are women; by the year 2010, it is estimated that one in three doctors will be female), more patients, both male and female, are beginning to select women doctors as their primary physicians. These patients seem to have sensed what studies have verified: Women physicians tend to spend more time with their patients, provide more information, and encourage their patients to discuss problems and ask questions.

How Important Are Communication Skills?

Many doctors disagree on the importance of a physician's communication skills, believing that it's far more important to have a skilled physician with no bedside manner than an adequate one with a pleasing personality. We suspect these doctors may be protesting too much. They themselves may be merely "good" doctors with no bedside manner. They also may not accept that healing entails far more than a correct diagnosis and treatment; strong communication skills enable a physician to reach out to a patient, offering understanding, comfort, and compassion that may help trigger an immune system to fight off disease and promote healing.

Why are communication skills so important? Because the patient-physician relationship depends on trust and understanding of one another. It must be a partnership. Patients who feel the doctor is empathetic and will take time to listen may open up, talk more freely, and give valuable clues that help the doctor make his or her diagnosis. These patients may feel more comfortable asking questions about treatment plans. This comfort level, in the long run, may make them more compliant, that is, more willing to follow the doctor's instructions about taking and completing a course of medication, exercising, losing weight, or even undergoing a painful procedure. These patients feel that their doctor really cares about them. (Studies show that patients with this type of open communication with their physicians are less likely to sue their doctors when problems do arise.)

In many cases, it is the *illusion* of spending more time with a patient, rather than actually spending more time, that creates this comfort level. The doctor sits down and listens to the patient, rather than edging toward the door or writing notes as the patient speaks. The physician maintains appropriate eye contact, and through body language (leaning forward, nodding, and so on, which often is more revealing than verbal cues) shows interest, compassion, and concern. Frequently, a physician will learn that what's bothering you is a painful relationship, a work problem, or just plain loneliness and a sense of not being needed. None of these symptoms require drugs with numerous and sometimes debilitating side effects or expensive, uncomfortable, invasive tests, only the sense that someone cares. Often, this was the treatment of choice for physicians of earlier days, who had little else with which to treat their patients.

Dr. John Connolly, author of *How to Find the Best Doctors, Hospitals, and HMOs for You and Your Family*, lists the following points to consider in selecting a physician:

- Medical education and specialized training
- Board (specialty) certification, which means taking additional training and passing specific arduous national written exams. (To verify that a physician is board certified, call the American Board of Medical Specialists at 1-800-776-CERT.)
- Hospital appointments and privileges
- Personality: Patient interaction and relationships
- Practice arrangements including billing, office hours, insurance, coverage by other doctors when out-of-town, ill, or otherwise unavailable
- History of problems or malpractice

At this writing, Massachusetts is the only state to release, at no charge, extensive information about physicians licensed by that state (call the Massachusetts Board of Registration in Medicine at (617) 727-0773 or 1-800-377-0550). Those in other states can get similar information free through the American Medical Association's Web site (http://www.ama-assn.org), or for $15 by contacting Medi-Net (http://www/askmedi.com), or through Public Citizen, an organization founded by consumer activist Ralph Nader, at (202) 588-1000.

HOSPITAL MEDICAL STAFF

Unless you're admitted through the emergency room, your personal physician (or surgeon) probably is the doctor who will actually admit you to the hospital, but he or she won't be the only one you'll see. Like rabbits, doctors tend to multiply once you're in the hospital, and their bills for "consulting" won't be asking for carrots in return.

You'll see more doctors (and doctors-in-training) in a teaching hospital, but you won't have to pay for all of them, only those called "attendings," who have been called in for a consult. In a private hospital, however, you pay for every physician your internist or family practitioner has asked to stop by to see you. The specialties vary, of course, depending on your medical problem.

Take as an example, the baffling "fever of unknown (or undetermined) origin," best known as "FUO." It is an unexplained fever that could be triggered by a variety of medical problems, some of them quite serious. FUO may be accompanied by chills. When your fever doesn't go away or keeps returning for several weeks, your cautious internist admits you to the hospital to prevent your becoming dehydrated and to conduct a few tests. You'll be X-rayed, scanned, have your blood, urine, and stool cultured, have your history taken and retaken, and be examined frequently. When no definite findings arise, your physician may call in an infectious disease expert, who prescribes more tests and possibly some medication. (Fifty percent of hospitalized FUOs are due to occult infections, including fungal infections, such as tuberculosis. Drug resistant TB is a major cause of infection and death in AIDS patients.) If the expert isn't sure what's wrong, your doctor may call in an oncologist, just to be sure you don't have some type of cancer. (At least one-fourth of all hospitalized FUOs are due to malignancies.) If you develop a bone abscess, an orthopaedic surgeon will be called in. When a rash also develops (perhaps because you're allergic to the laundry detergent in the hospital sheets), a dermatologist drops by. If your head begins to hurt, your doctor may fear meningitis and ask for a neurology consult.

If you're admitted to a teaching hospital with FUO, you may have your history taken and first be examined by a PA (physician's assistant) or by an intern, now also called PGY1 (post graduate year #1).

Doctors in their first year of training after graduation from medical school used to be called "interns." (Don't confuse that with "internist," an internal medicine specialist who is "trained in the essentials of primary care internal medicine, which incorporates an understanding of disease prevention, wellness, substance abuse, mental health, and effective treatment of common problems of the eyes, ears, skin, nervous system, and reproductive organs."[1]) Although interns are still called that in many hospitals, the usual term is now "residents," whether it is the physician's first, second, or third year. "A physician's residency training begins after he or she successfully completes medical school, and it can last anywhere from three to seven years, with five years being the minimum for the surgical specialties."[2]

Don't write off residents as being less qualified, however. Although they may not have as much actual hands-on experience as a physician who has been in practice for many years, these

---

[1] *The American Board of Medical Specialties, Which Medical Specialist for You (Evanston, IL: 1995)*, 12.
[2] *The American College of Surgeons, Modern Surgery: A Profession of Challenge and Opportunity (Chicago: 1991)*, 17.

doctors may be more conscientious because they *are* new to the profession. They have just learned the newest procedures for helping patients and have fewer bad habits to break. Many of these men and women are more used to listening to their patients (what isn't said as well as what is), have more patience, and have yet to develop the hard protective shell that so many physicians wrap around themselves.

As a caveat, however, residents usually will order more tests and other procedures because (1) they probably have never been patients themselves and (2) they want technological backup as reassurance that they are not missing something in their diagnosis or treatment of your condition.

Regardless of the impeccable credentials of any or all of the parade of medical mavens who stop by your bedside, remember that you are the most important part of the team. Don't just lie passively in your hospital bed and nod mutely as the doctor talks to you. Offer information if no one thinks to ask. Your being on a camping trip just before you began to run a fever might offer important clues to your FUO. You could have had contaminated drinking water or been bitten by a rat, flea, or other insect. Don't do what one woman did and think, "He's the doctor. He should figure out what's wrong."

Ask questions, too. Your life may depend on it.

- What is your name? Repeat your name to the doctor as well to be sure he or she hasn't wandered into the wrong room.

- What is your specialty?

- Why has my doctor asked you to see me?

- How many of these procedures (surgical or otherwise invasive) have you done?

- Will you actually be doing the procedure or merely supervising it?

- What are the side effects of this procedure?

- What is the cost of your services?

If you don't have someone in the room with you to provide a second set of ears, turn on your tape recorder if you thought to bring one. If not, take notes. It not only puts the physician on notice that what is being said is "for the record," but it also helps clear up confusion if you can't remember what you heard. It also defends your position if you get a bill from a doctor who claims to have seen you, but didn't, a practice that has occurred with elderly patients who are covered by Medicare and who often don't see what has been paid out by the government until after the fact.

Mark the tape or notebook with the date, time, and the physician's name and give it to someone for safe keeping. Remember that you are the consumer and must take responsibility for your own body. Ask questions; there are no "stupid" ones.

If you don't like a particular doctor's attitude or lack of communication skills, notice that his or her voice is slurred, or smell alcohol, tell your personal physician or the attending physician that you want someone else. If that doctor tries to talk you out of changing, ask why. Perhaps they are personal friends. Demand to speak to the patient advocate or if the hospital doesn't have one, the hospital administrator.

Medicine must be a partnership with the physician accepting a role that is far more than just that of a technician. You are not an automobile coming into the shop for a tune-up. You are a precious human being, placing your life and well-being in the hands of another, and deserve to be treated as such. As Melvin Konner, M.D., writes in his book, *Medicine at the Crossroads: The Crisis in Health Care,* "Almost every patient needs to believe that his or her doctor really cares, at least a little; that the doctor's effort is a serious one, mobilizing powerful resources on the patient's behalf; and that if the treatment fails, it will not be because the doctor omitted some reasonable approach that might have worked—not, in other words, because the doctor did not care."[3]

If you don't like or trust the physicians involved in your care or feel that there is a communication problem, you may be compromising your ability to enjoy a successful recovery. The mind-body connection is all powerful. When you put your health or that of a loved one in someone else's hands, you need confidence, trust, and the belief that the healer cares about you and your needs, and is willing to accept you as an active member of the healing team.

Become knowledgeable in your own medical care. What you don't know *can* hurt you. Check your local library or medical library for information. Ask your doctor for booklets and other literature pertaining to your medical condition. Contact computer bulletin board support groups and access computerized data banks such as the National Library of Medicine's MEDLINE which contains data from more than 3,500 medical journals. The World Wide Web probably contains all the medical information you want or need to know. If you don't know how to use a modem, contact your local high school or college for the name of a reliable computer whiz.

Specialists

Surgeons are probably the first medical specialists that come to mind, as many people entering a hospital are there for surgery. But even this specialty is subdivided and includes the following:

- *General surgeons* perform operations on almost any area of the body. They also may be board certified in specific subspecialties, such as general vascular surgery, pediatric surgery, surgical critical care, and hand

[3] *Melvin Konner, M.D.*, Medicine at the Crossroads: The Crisis in Health Care *(New York: Pantheon Books, 1993), 13.*

surgery. Each of these areas of expertise requires additional training.

- *Colon and rectal surgeons* deal surgically with, but are not limited to, the intestinal tract, colon, rectum, and anal canal, as well as organs and tissue affected by intestinal disease. In addition to surgery, these specialists perform endoscopic procedures to detect and treat conditions of the bowel lining.

- *General vascular surgeons* operate on surgical disorders of the blood vessels.

- *Thoracic surgeons* perform surgery on the chest, including treating coronary artery disease; cancers of the lung, esophagus, and chest wall; abnormalities of the great vessels and heart valves; congenital anomalies; and diseases of the diaphragm.

- *Neurosurgeons* perform surgery on the brain, brain stem, skull, spine, spinal cord, and nerves.

- *Oncology surgeons* operate on patients suffering from various forms of cancer.

- *Otolaryngologists* for ear, nose, and throat. The otolaryngologist head and neck surgeon is popularly referred to as an ENT, and has been trained to care for patients with diseases and disorders affecting the ears, respiratory and upper alimentary systems and related structures, and the head and neck in general.

- *Plastic surgeons* perform cosmetic and reconstructive surgery dealing with the repair, reconstruction, or replacement of physical defects of form or function involving the skin, musculoskeletal system, cranio-maxillofacial structures, hand, extremities, breast and trunk, and external genitalia. Often the plastic surgeon will be in the operating room with the oncology surgeon, standing by to reconstruct a breast or other area once the cancer has been removed.

- *Gynecologists* deal with disorders affecting the female reproductive system.

- *Orthopaedic surgeons* operate on problems relating to the skeletal and muscular system. There also are surgeons who deal only with the hand and wrist.

- *Pediatric surgeons* operate on children, from premature infants and newborns to teenagers.

- *Anesthesiologists*, although not surgeons, are medical doctors with four or more years of postgraduate training and are a vital part of any surgical team. They administer drugs to render the patient unconscious or numb at the surgical site, monitor breathing and pain response, and interact with the surgeon throughout the procedure. Anesthesiologists also may deal with pain control after surgery.

Certified registered nurse anesthetists (CRNA) also administer anesthetics, working with or under the supervision of the anesthesiologist. The CRNAs are not medical doctors, but are registered nurses with a minimum of two years of specialized graduate-level education in anesthesia. They also must pass a national certification exam and complete a continuing education and recertification program every two years.

All these subspecialties have their pediatric counterparts. Children are not "little adults." Their reactions to anesthesia and surgery itself differ from those of grown-ups. Request a pediatric specialist—especially a pediatric surgeon—whenever possible for your child.

Nursing Staff

Hospital nurses play a variety of roles. They are the teachers of information, the caregivers, the facilitators of the physician's orders. They are professional men and women, and are graduates of one of three types of programs: a four-year baccalaureate nursing program, a two-year associate degree program from a junior college (the scope of practice is more defined to hospital-based nursing), or a three-year diploma nursing program from a hospital-based nursing program (currently being phased out other than in rural or isolated areas).

According to Lois W. Lowry, R.N., D.N.Sc., Associate Professor and Interim Associate Dean of the Baccalaureate Program, University of South Florida College of Nursing, "Registered nurses have independent, interdependent, and dependent functions. Independent functions are those activities considered to be within the nurse's scope of diagnosis and treatment, including comprehensive assessments of patients (physical, psychosocial, spiritual, and emotional development) and implementation of measures designed to motivate, teach, and support the patient and family. These actions do not require a physician's order in that they treat the responses to illness such as teaching diet, insulin administration, and skin care to diabetics after the diagnosis has been made by a physician. Interdependent functions are carried out in collaboration with other health-care providers such as physical therapists, occupational therapists, and dietitians, just to mention a few. They also have supervisory responsibility for ancillary personnel such as LPNs, technicians, aides, and others. Dependent functions are those based upon physician's orders."

Nurses also act as conduits between physician and patient, to assure optimum results. Typical functions include listening to patients' fears and concerns and helping to reassure them; explaining procedures; administering medications, securing tubes and drains; assisting with personal care; applying and changing dressings; and watching for any emotional or physical signs that might signal drug allergy, worsening of a condition, or new symptoms.

The nurse is a teacher, instructing family and friends as well as the patient about ways to make the patient more comfortable. He or she teaches new mothers, patients learning to live with disabilities or with chronic conditions, as well as preventive care. The main emphasis of nursing is health promotion and disease prevention. Nursing is wellness focused, not illness focused, which is the doctor's domain. Nurses promote wellness and achievement of wellness after illness strikes. Said Dr. Lowry, "One can always delegate others to do caregiver functions, but the teaching role requires the more extensive educational preparation that an R.N. receives." A nurse must be able to quickly assess not only a patient's condition, but also the dynamics of a family unit, in order to determine the best way to offer education and emotional support to the patient and his or her family.

Fifty years ago, new mothers were kept in the hospital for two weeks and treated to backrubs and careful instruction on how to care for themselves and their newborn. It was usually a registered nurse who performed these tasks. This was an important function. Often the registered nurse was able to assess a potential problem—an infant's jaundice, a mother's cracked nipples, or poor parenting technique, and arrange for treatment before serious harm was done. It also offered the time for a nurse to get to know each patient as a human being rather than a number. Fortunately, since legislation was passed in 1996, it is now illegal for insurance companies to force hospitals to discharge a mother less than twenty-four hours after giving birth as had been the previous practice. It is now, as it should be, a decision to be made between the mother and her physician.

This need to know a patient is more than a nicety. The nurse is responsible for issuing the medications prescribed by your physician, but also must observe the effects of these drugs. Everyone reacts differently to medications and a nurse who is knowledgeable about the effects can quickly surmise when a patient is having side effects and react quickly to help. Also, because they see their patients more frequently than physicians, nurses may be able to learn things about a patient that could affect the healing process—such as a depression, fear of going home to responsibility, or anxiety. Even a procedure as seemingly simple as a bed bath should be done by an R.N. or an L.P.N. because he or she is trained to notice the beginning of a bedsore (which can become infected and could cause death) and to otherwise observe the patient's physical and emotional reactions.

Your perception of your care and the actual quality of your care rest in the hands of these overworked, often underpaid, and underrecognized men and women. With financial pressures often the force driving a hospital, many trained and experienced registered nurses have been replaced by licensed practical nurses, who may be equally dedicated to their patients but who have not had the same education as a registered nurse. In many hospitals the person (usually female) caring for you is not even an L.P.N., but a nurse's aide or nurse technician.

Don't assume the "nurse" caring for you is a registered nurse; ask.

Technicians

This category is an ever-growing one as new technologies enter the medical field with startling rapidity. Unfortunately, many technicians receive training only in how to carry out a particular procedure, with little if any education in how to handle people, especially frightened ones. They may have no expertise in dealing with the unique problems of the elderly, those who are hearing or visually impaired, or the pediatric population.

One of the most familiar technicians is the person in the X-ray department. He or she positions you on the table or in front of an X-ray plate, tells you to take a deep breath, and then scurries behind a protective wall to take the picture. If you're lucky, the technician remembers to tell you when you can breathe again. Don't hesitate to request a lead apron to protect parts of your body

Always tell the X-ray technician if there is any possibility you could be pregnant if he or she forgets to ask.

(especially your reproductive organs) not being subjected to radiation if the X-ray technician has forgotten to provide it.

The medical technician who pops into your hospital room with a metal carrier of clanging glass vials is called a phlebotomist. He or she ties a flexible rubber cord around your upper arm to make your veins stand out, then, with a syringe, draws blood to be used for various testing procedures. Usually a vein in the crook of your arm is useable, although sometimes the phlebotomist will have to use a finger, a vein in your foot, or one in another area of your body.

If your veins are fragile, hard to find, or the patient is a child or elderly person, ask the phlebotomist to use smaller needles to draw the blood. After two or three unsuccessful attempts, both you and the technician are going to be nervous. Under this circumstance, you have the right to insist on a replacement to draw the necessary blood or to insert the IV needle.

If your arms are bruised by constant drawing of blood samples, you have the right to demand just one bloodletting a day, unless the physician ordering the extra specimen can tell you a medical reason why he or she couldn't use blood from the one drawn earlier.

Your physician may order an electrocardiogram (EKG), which is a noninvasive monitoring of your heart's electrical function. The EKG technician will put an ointment on your chest, leg, and other parts of your body and place electrodes on these areas. Wires are connected from the electrodes to a small portable EKG machine. You'll feel no sensation while this test is being performed, so just rest quietly while your heart does all the work. Afterwards, the technician will remove the wires, wipe off the salve, and leave, frequently without saying more than a few words to you.

Therapists

You may be seen by any number of therapists in the hospital, depending on your medical problem. Each type of therapist has received specific education and training and performs a definite function.

The *respiratory therapist* is a trained specialist who is state certified and whose job it is to help you to improve lung function after surgery, disease, or a long confinement in bed. This can help prevent pneumonia from setting in. He or she may give you explicit exercises to perform. Follow these instructions to the letter and don't think you're fooling anyone by "cheating." You're the one who needs them to get better, not the therapist. The respiratory therapist also may have you breathe into a machine to help you take deeper breaths. If you're concerned about how the tubing on the breathing machine was cleaned before your using it, express these or any other concerns to the therapist.

The *speech therapist* holds a degree in that specialty and is also licensed by your state. He or she helps you regain and improve communication skills and relearn to swallow after surgery or a stroke.

The *physical therapist,* a certified specialist, will come to your bedside to help you regain and strengthen muscle tone to prevent your joints from stiffening and to ward off blood clots, and to improve coordination after surgery, accident, illness, or stroke. If you need a cane, crutches, or have a new artificial limb, this individual will teach you how to use it and care for it. Later, if you are still in the hospital, you will be brought to the physical therapy (PT) department where there are mats, balls, and other equipment to help further your rehabilitation. Physical therapists use active exercise, hydrotherapy, visualization, and massage, as well as other techniques.

Occupational therapists aid with rehabilitation efforts by teaching methods for improving activities of daily living (ADL). This incorporates a variety of techniques including special equipment such as eating utensils that fit over the hand, rather than being held with your fingers, a sock holder to help slide the foot into the socks, and a model kitchen at wheelchair height or with special fittings for faucets and drawers.

Play therapists, also called child life specialists, use toys, arts and crafts, and other activities to help children express their fears and anxieties more fully. Play therapy helps children deal with issues of self-esteem, separation, and loss of control. Medical play, in which children act out fears using dolls, medical masks, syringes, and other hospital equipment, helps children become more comfortable with their hospital experience.

Creative arts therapists include music, art, and dance/movement therapy to help patients who are depressed, chronically ill, or recovering from an illness. Arts and crafts—especially working with clay, paints, or chalk—are especially effective with those who are unable or unwilling to express their emotions verbally. Music and movement also aid the ability to tap into emotions that are difficult to express verbally. Needlepoint and weaving encourage range-of-motion exercise, work hand muscles, help eye control, and offer a myriad of additional benefits

Horticultural therapists are found in some hospitals fortunate enough to have space for gardening. Since 1959, the Howard A. Rusk Institute of Rehabilitation at NYU Medical Center in New York has had a garden for patients, not only for enjoyment, but also to aid their rehabilitation. It encourages their use of small, fine hand movements as well as improves balance.

Psychotherapists may be psychologists, psychiatrists, social workers, creative arts therapists, or any skilled professionals who focus on establishing a relationship with the patient to accomplish therapeutical goals. You don't have to be "crazy" to need to talk to such a professional. Just being in a hospital is stressful enough; most people need someone to talk to about their anxieties and fears. You may not want to let your family members know that you're frightened or worried about the outcome of your medical situation. If your physician doesn't suggest a consultation with a psychotherapist and you feel you'd like to talk to one, ask.

Social Workers

Social workers are trained professionals, usually on the hospital staff, who help to coordinate services and communication between the various departments of the hospital. They provide counseling, do crisis interventions, and guide the patient and family through the maze of paperwork and forms.

Social workers not only act as the patient advocate while the patient is hospitalized, but also are knowledgeable of the services available in your particular community, such as home health care, respite care, nursing homes, assisted living facilities, Meals on Wheels, and so on. They can direct you or your family member to a service agency as needed for family problems; availability of equipment such as hospital bed, bedside commode, or wheelchair; economic needs; ongoing outside counseling; and so on.

Usually, social workers will contact you upon arrival to ascertain your needs before discharge. If not, seek them out. You're wandering in a strange, new land when you're in a hospital. You don't have to do it alone. The social worker is an educated guide. Take that helping hand.

Clergy

Many hospitals, especially those with a religious affiliation, have a full-time chaplain or department head of what is called "pastoral care." The chaplain may call on you to see if you have a personal priest, minister, or rabbi. He or she can care for your spiritual needs, if you prefer.

Pastoral care offers more than spiritual support, however. These members of the clergy also provide counseling, a nonmedical shoulder to lean on, and sometimes, a non-judgmental ear for you to vent your emotions. They don't need to be of your religious persuasion to be supportive.

Dietitians

A registered dietitian is a trained professional who has received a bachelor's degree in nutrition or a related field from an accredited school. He or she has performed a required internship and passed a national exam. Ideally, the dietitian should meet with you shortly after you are admitted to the hospital to discuss your food plan while you are in the hospital. Be sure to tell the dietitian if there are any foods you dislike or to which you have allergies. Although it should be noted on your chart, mistakes do happen, so stay alert.

Orderlies

Orderlies are also known as transporters, probably because they transport people and things. Some are friendly and chatty, to help patients relax. Others move you along without speaking as though you were the sheet you're (almost) covered with. If the silence bothers you, start talking.

If the orderly is taking your child or an elderly loved one somewhere, tag along. Otherwise, the patient may be lined up in the hall outside the X-ray or procedure room and left alone. It can be frightening, even if you aren't eight or eighty.

Housekeeping Staff

What does the housekeeping staff have to do with your health in the hospital? A great deal, actually.

Hospitals overflow with germs and sick people, a dangerous and sometimes fatal combination. Weakened immune systems are vulnerable to the smorgasbord of bacteria thriving within the hospital environment. In fact, infection is the most common cause of death in cancer patients who were or recently had been hospitalized.

Bacteria enter our bodies through urinary catheters, IV lines, respiratory therapy tubing, surgical incisions, non-sterile dressings, and non-sterilized dishes and glassware. Or we ingest bacteria simply by breathing in the air from other sick people directly or through the air-conditioning/heating vents. Larger hospitals and teaching hospitals have higher nosocomial infection rates (hospital-acquired infections) than smaller facilities because they tend to deal with sicker people and greater numbers of people.

> ☞ Do your part to help minimize infection by washing your hands often, whether you're the patient or a family member. Keep your hands away from your eyes, nose, mouth, and the surgical site. Contact the housekeeping department immediately if the hospital room seems dirty or you run out of soap or paper towels.

Many of us, overfed on antibiotics prescribed by physicians who felt (often because of *our* demands) that they had to give us something, are now faced with bacteria that are resistant to antibiotics, rendering us defenseless against these nosocomial infections.

Although many of these infections are airborne and settle within the respiratory system, urinary tract, and incision area, they can be controlled to some degree by constant vigilance by the housekeeping crew. This includes disinfecting door handles, telephone receivers, television remotes, and bathrooms; removing dirty linens and food trays promptly; and emptying wastepaper baskets regularly.

Volunteers

Volunteers save hospitals thousands of dollars by running errands, working in the gift shop, delivering flowers and mail, and transporting patients. However, their lack of training in regard to health measures may be hazardous to patients. Few hospitals train their volunteer staff to take precautions when suffering from a cough or sore throat; afflicted with sinus, urinary tract, or skin infections; or carrying even a slight fever. In their quest to do good and not let the hospital down by skipping their shift, many well-meaning but slightly ill volunteers visit room after room, bringing bacteria in with the mail and germs with the geraniums.

CHAPTER 4

Hospital Hazards: How to Avoid Infections, Drug Errors, and Surgical Mistakes

"You need to go to the hospital." When we hear those words from our physician, our perception often is that we are surrendering ourselves (or a family member) to the loving care of substitute mommies in an all-protective environment where we will be treated for our disease or disorder and made well again.

The reality is that, according to a study by Harvard School of Public Health, hospital-related errors in treatment kill an estimated 180,000 Americans each year, and injure hundreds of thousands more. According to a report in the January 22–29, 1997 issue of *JAMA,* three new studies show that adverse drug events (i.e., bad reactions to drugs or errors in prescribing them) alone occur in 6.5 percent of hospitalized patients and may account for up to 140,000 deaths per year. (For comparison, U.S. deaths over a ten-year period in Vietnam were 57,000.) What's more, 5 to 10 percent (or more, depending on which particular study is used) of hospitalized patients will develop an infection they didn't have when they came into the hospital. These infections bring with them added discomfort and pain; extra, often invasive, procedures; lengthier hospital stays; additional expense; and, sometimes, even death. Unfortunately, these infections are so common that they even have their own name: nosocomial infections. It means "hospital-acquired" infections.

NOSOCOMIAL INFECTIONS

Hand Washing Is Essential

In 1860, a Hungarian doctor named Ignaz Phillipp Semmelweis wrote and published *The Etiology, Concept and Prophylaxis of Childbirth Fever,* in which he declared that doctors were spreading puerperal fever (known as childbirth fever) by not washing their hands between patient examinations. During his lifetime, Semmelweis was mocked for his ideas by his peers. But in 1865, the year of Semmelweis' death, a British surgeon, Joseph Lister, performed his first antiseptic surgery. Shortly thereafter, following sterile procedures became the norm throughout civilized medical communities.

Sad, then, that despite this knowledge, gained through the sacrifice of many women's lives, anywhere from 80,000 to 100,000 hospitalized patients in America die every year from these often preventable infections. Amazingly, among the major contributors to the spread of these infections are doctors themselves. (There is even a name for doctor-created disorders: iatrogenic disease.) One of the most common causes? Depressingly simple. The failure to wash their hands. (Drug reactions and errors are another major cause of iatrogenic disease.)

According to a study conducted at two general pediatric clinics of two medical schools, 51 percent of physicians did not wash their hands just before a patient encounter. Of this number, fewer than 10 percent washed their hands immediately after examining the patient and going on to check another.

It's a common sight in a hospital to see physicians making rounds, checking one patient after the other without bothering to wash their hands with antibacterial soap between patients. In one case, we observed an orthopaedic surgeon remove the bloody dressings from a patient who had recently undergone knee replacement surgery without washing his hands or putting on gloves. He tossed the soiled dressing on the patient's bedside table (where her lunch tray would soon rest), examined the incision, then expertly re-dressed the wound. He answered a few questions, then patted his patient on her shoulder and left the room, headed for the next patient. It was no surprise to hear later that this patient's wound became infected, which required additional medical attention and extra expense, and resulted in a delayed recovery period.

Ask physicians, nurses, and technicians to wash their hands before examining you or beginning a procedure. If they're wearing gloves and remove them after doing a procedure, such as inserting a bronchial or urinary catheter, request that they wash their hands before further examining you.

Equipment Should Be Washed, Too

Although the Centers for Disease Control in Atlanta and the American Hospital Association encourage hand washing by doctors and nurses after patient contact, the recommendation is often ignored. However, while the failure to wash hands is a major cause of nosocomial and iatrogenic infections in hospitals, there are numerous others. Equipment, even as basic as the stethoscope or the otoscope (the device through which the doctor looks into your ears), can transfer harmful bacteria when it comes in contact with patient after patient without being cleaned between usage (unless it has disposable shields).

According to a study of 150 emergency medical personnel conducted by researchers at Butterworth Hospital in Grand Rapids, Michigan, and Michigan State University in East Lansing, stethoscopes are infrequently or never cleaned by their users. About 48 percent of those interviewed said they disinfected their stethoscopes daily or weekly by wiping them with an alcohol swab. Thirty-seven percent admitted to cleaning them only once a month. Seven percent cleaned them once a year and another 7 percent said they never disinfected them. Nurses appeared to be more diligent about cleaning their stethoscopes than physicians. Yet when the researchers cultured the stethoscopes for bacteria, they discovered 89 percent contaminated with staphylococci, which can cause skin infections, and 19 percent with Staphylococcus aureus, a more virulent form of the bacteria, which can be extremely dangerous for someone with an open wound or a compromised immune system.[1] The AMA brief from *Internal Medicine,* January 15, 1997, referred to staph-contaminated stethoscopes as "killer stethoscopes."

Improper cleaning or total lack of cleaning of other instruments and equipment, such as infusion pumps, contaminated endoscopes and bronchoscopes, or hemodialysis equipment, is another source of nosocomial infection. Infection also can be introduced with the use of catheters, tubing inserted either into a vein for the purpose of introducing hydration or medications or into the bladder to drain off urine. (In fact, urinary catheters were found to be responsible for more than 40 percent of all nosocomial infections.)

Intensive Care Unit Hazards

Even patients in the areas set aside for those whose conditions require constant medical monitoring, such as the intensive care units (ICUs) and coronary care units (CCUs), are not exempt from

[1] *Adapted from an article in the "Quality Watch" column of* Hospitals & Health Networks, *5 November 1995, p. 13. Study based on research at Butterworth Hospital, Grand Rapids, MI, and Michigan State University, East Lansing.*

hospital-acquired infections. In fact, they are in greater danger from it, especially from pneumonia, with the incidence varying from 7 percent to more than 40 percent of patients in intensive care units. In addition, these people are also most vulnerable to respiratory tract infections, urinary tract infections, and sepsis or bloodstream infections. In fact, as reported in the January 11, 1995, edition of *The Journal of the American Medical Association* (*JAMA*), sepsis has been reported to be the most common cause of death in noncoronary ICUs.[2] It's really not surprising. The patients in these units are at high risk. They are extremely ill and have weakened immune systems. They are bedded in close quarters next to other critically ill patients. They suffer from heightened stress from fear and anxiety. They experience sleep deprivation because the overhead lights are always on; there is a cacophony of clatter, conversation, and confusion; and they are constantly being monitored and/or cared for because of their precarious conditions. No wonder their immune system is vulnerable to infection.

Although these patients are cared for by highly trained professionals, the staff is often overworked. Some take on two shift assignments and many suffer from potential burnout due to the stress of working in such a highly charged atmosphere. Sterile procedures, even those as basic as hand washing, are often forgotten or omitted due to the pressures inherent in the intensive care environment. Personnel with colds or staph-related boils, carbuncles, or pimples can easily spread infection to patients through contact with towels, dressings, and other contaminated articles. And frequently, if the number of patients (census) is particularly high, the full-time staff in these intensive care facilities may be augmented by nurses from temporary agencies who have limited experience working in an ICU.

For all these reasons, we urge you to get out of the ICU as quickly as possible, for your health's sake. According to a March 20,

---

[2]M.S. Neiderman and A. M. Fein, "Sepsis Syndrome, The Adult Respiratory Distress Syndrome, and Nosocomial Pneumonia: A Common Clinical Sequence," Clinical Chest Medicine *11 (1990): 633–656.*

1996, article in *JAMA,* patients sick enough to be admitted into the ICU "have nosocomial infection rates that are as much as five to 10 times higher than those in the general wards."[3]

Operating rooms (ORs), supposedly the bastions of bacteria-free surroundings, can also be hazardous to a patient's well-being. Sterile equipment can easily become contaminated. Physicians, technicians, and nurses may cough or sneeze even through their protective masks, wipe their noses with gloved hands, change stations on the radio with gloved hands, or otherwise break the sterile field. Anesthesiologists and/or nurse anesthetists may fail to wear gloves while performing various presurgical procedures. Sales representatives of new orthopaedic appliances, despite regulations forbidding it, often come into the OR to supervise or oversee a surgeon using the device. Even the media may be invited into the OR to observe, often garbed in protective scrubs, foot covering, and masks, but still carrying bacteria-covered cameras, microphones, pens, and notebooks to record what they are witnessing.

A study in the May 9, 1996, issue of *JAMA* revealed that "wound infections are common and serious complications of anesthesia and surgery." The investigators learned that "In patients undergoing colon surgery, the risk of such an infection ranges from 3 to 22 percent, depending on such factors as the length of surgery and underlying medical problems."[4]

MISUSE OF ANTIBIOTICS

Misuse and overuse of antibiotics, especially for viral infections (which are seldom affected by antibiotics), have enabled many types of bacteria to become resistant to so-called "miracle drugs." This antibiotic resistance has caused serious and sometimes fatal

[3] Jean-Yves Fagon, M.D. et al., "Nosocomial Pneumonia and Mortality Among Patients in Intensive Care Units," JAMA 275, no. 11 (20 March 1996): 866.
[4] D. H. Culver et al., "Surgical Wound Infection Rates by Wound Class, Operative Procedure, and Patient Risk Index," American Journal of Medicine 91 (1991): 152S–157S.

☞ Never urge your doctor to give you an antibiotic; your condition may not require it. Some physicians reluctantly prescribe antibiotics at their patient's request because they feel the patient (or the family) may feel nothing is being done if there's no prescription for an antibiotic. Always ask, "Do I need an antibiotic? Will it treat my infection?" If the answer is, "Well, it can't hurt . . . ," refuse it. It *can* hurt.

---

problems, especially to those who are sickest—patients in the ICUs and the cancer wards. All patients with compromised immune systems, those who are critically ill, the very young, and the elderly can die from infections recently so easily cured. Surprisingly, even previously healthy people are known to have died from these antibiotic-resistant infections. And the number of this type of infection is growing. A report from the Centers for Disease Control and Prevention in Atlanta (CDC) said infections with the bacteria strain called vancomycin-resistant enterococcus (VRE) have increased from 0.3 percent in 1989 to 7.9 percent at most recent count, in 1993.

According to the CDC, metropolitan Atlanta has experienced a 35 percent rise in cases of drug-resistant streptococcus pneumonia over the last two years. They also reported a 1996 outbreak in a New York hospital of multi-drug-resistant tuberculosis involving patients with acquired immunodeficiency syndrome (AIDS). It raised concerns about a potentially fatal illness that could be easily transmitted and was potentially untreatable.

IATROGENIC DISEASE

An iatrogenic disease is one that is caused by the physician. It may be an infection or condition caused by a doctor's actions, ranging from a physician performing a procedure that makes things worse rather than better to the doctor's causing a problem where there was none before.

Iatrogenic illnesses result from procedures including wrong-sited surgery; approximately half of the hysterectomies performed, which are unnecessary; the prescribing of the tranquilizer thalidomide, which caused babies to be born with flipper-like arms; radiation for hemorrhoids and acne; and the giving of blood-clotting substances that contain the hepatitis A virus to hemophiliacs. (Until recent years, hemophiliacs also were subjected to batches of contaminated clotting factors that contained the hepatitis B and C viruses as well as the AIDS virus.) Iatrogenic illnesses are also caused by medications.

Iatrogenic problems are, in addition, those created when a physician mistakenly treats a patient for the wrong illness; when a surgeon attempts a procedure he or she has not fully mastered; or when complications develop because the physician wasn't prepared for an emergency situation.

Many human errors can lead and have led to wrong-sited surgery. The surgeon picks up another patient's X rays before operating or films are inserted backwards into the view box in the OR; a nursing aide shaves or preps the wrong side before surgery; someone else's surgery is canceled so you are moved up in the operating room order and nobody removes the other patient's documentation; or nurses drape the wrong side.

Physicians with contagious illnesses have been known to pass them along to their patients. During 1991 and 1992, a young physician being trained in thoracic surgery unknowingly infected nineteen of his patients with the extremely infectious hepatitis B virus (HBV). Another report described five patients contracting hepatitis C (HCV) after having open-heart surgery done by a cardiac surgeon infected with hepatitis C.

It is estimated that 1,900 American surgeons today are infected with hepatitis B, which can be fatal. According to investigators of the Centers for Disease Control and Prevention in Atlanta, the outbreak in the first case mentioned above could have been prevented if the doctor had been inoculated with the hepatitis B vaccine. In fact, with today's ever-increasing incidence of hepatitis, we believe that *all* operating personnel—indeed, all health-care providers—should be vaccinated for hepatitis B.

Although a surgeon's use of gloves and masks while operating offers some protection to you, the patient, it obviously isn't fool-proof. Surgical equipment and bone fragments can cause pinpoint tears in gloves that are not visible to the naked eye. It's likely that sterile gloves and masks probably do more to protect the surgeon and operating room staff from the bacteria in *your* system than the other way around.

Hepatitis also can be contracted through a blood transfusion. Most of us worry about getting the HIV virus through a blood transfusion. But since 1985, when all donated blood began being checked for the AIDS virus, the chances of contracting hepatitis is more common and causes far more fatalities.

According to an article in *American Health* by Andrew G. Kadar, an anesthesiologist at Cedars-Sinai Medical Center in Los Angeles, testing by blood banks for hepatitis B began in 1971 and for hepatitis C in 1990. Both of these viruses can destroy liver cells and could lead to liver cancer and death. Although present testing methods have reduced the chance of being exposed to these viruses through a transfusion (1 in 3,300 units for hepatitis C

Before selecting a particular surgeon to operate on you or a family member, ask if he or she has been inoculated against hepatitis B. Also, be concerned if the surgeon has an outbreak of pimples or boils on his or her face or any sign of an infection. These may be a sign of a persistent staph infection. You may be "fertile soil," more prone to catching this type of infection, which could make you critically ill or could prove fatal.

and 1 in 200,000 units for hepatitis B),[5] Dr. Kadar and other experts encourage patients undergoing surgery that may require a blood transfusion to stockpile their own for possible use. This procedure, called autologous transfusion, requires prospective patients to donate one unit per week for four to six weeks before surgery. Ask your surgeon about the possibility of your utilizing autologous transfusions if you're having elective surgery.

Sometimes, it may be difficult to get blood from a patient's veins without the vessels collapsing. In these cases, a family member or close friend with the same blood type (known to be disease-free) may offer to donate blood.

JUDGMENT AND DIAGNOSTIC ERRORS

Errors in judgment and diagnosis can harm a patient. Researchers affix much of the blame for this type of mistake on physicians' passive reliance on technology and objective laboratory reports, rather than trusting their powers of observation—what they see, feel, and hear for themselves.

A study by researchers from Baptist Memorial Hospital and the University of Tennessee College of Medicine and reported in the *JAMA* revealed that heart attacks were misdiagnosed 47 percent of the time. A Harvard hospital study detailed in the *New England Journal of Medicine* showed that 10 percent of all patients who had died *might have lived* if they had received the correct diagnosis. In some categories of disease, the misdiagnosis figures were as high as 24 percent.[6]

A physician's adult daughter suffered from headaches and was diagnosed with a benign brain cyst. The first neurologist who examined the girl said, "Rip it out. It will only grow larger."

His partner disagreed. "Let's wait and see what happens."

---

[5]*Andrew G. Kadar, M.D., "How Safe Is Our Blood Supply?"* American Health (*June 1996): 78–79, 105.*
[6]*Charles B. Inlander and Ed Weiner,* Take This Book to the Hospital with You (*Allentown, PA: People's Medical Society, 1993), 141.*

> Always ask for a second opinion or second reading of a laboratory report if the original report subjects you to surgery or other invasive procedures, a possibly toxic drug regimen, or painful treatments. Pay for the charges yourself if your insurance won't cover it, although most insurance policies now pay for second opinions. People have died unnecessarily simply because they hesitated to ask for a second opinion because their insurance didn't pay for it. Even if you have to borrow the money to pay your bill, you'll have a longer lifetime in which to pay it back.

In frustration, the father took his daughter to yet another neurologist. The third specialist studied the scans and suggested, "Let's operate and put in a shunt."

The father and his daughter discussed the options and selected the first neurologist's partner's decision to wait and see what happened. Six months later, when the scans were repeated, there was no sign of enlargement of the cyst. "What would have happened," the father asked the first physician's partner, "if we had gone with your partner's diagnosis and let him operate?"

"Your daughter would have had an unnecessary operation," he answered.

Drug, Surgical, and Other "Human Errors"

Regardless of the depth to which medical technology has entered the field of medicine, human beings are still involved. And being human, they make mistakes. Human error, caused by fatigue, haste, lack of focus due to personal problems, over-reliance on the "infallibility" of technology, carelessness, and just plain old ignorance, is responsible for most, although not all, of the drug, surgical, and other human errors. The remaining chapters will describe how these mistakes happen and what you can do to prevent them.

> ☛ While you obviously can't give a nurse the day off to rest up because he or she was up all night with a sick child, you can remain watchful and on the alert for mistakes that may arise because the nurse is exhausted. Be sympathetic if the nurse seems hurried and harried. But at the same time, ask him or her to double-check the dosage of the drug being handed to you, especially if it looks different from what you've been taking. Fatigue can create errors.

In Florida, a respiratory therapist, just returning from a six-week maternity leave and apparently exhausted by the demands of her new infant, walked into the wrong patient's room the first hour she was on duty. According to a hospital spokesman, she failed to check the patient's wrist identification band and turned off his ventilator rather than the one hooked up to the dying patient next door. The unlucky seventy-seven-year-old patient was recovering from earlier surgery. He had a tracheotomy and could neither speak nor make a noise when the ventilator was removed. The man suffered a cardiac arrest and died about half an hour after the therapy technician had disconnected him.

Two Wisconsin women died after a technician at the same medical laboratory, fatigued from reading more than twice the number of slides recommended by the American Society of Cytology, misread their Pap tests as negative (normal) rather than positive. By the time either woman's cervical cancer was discovered, it was too advanced for a cure. Both died of their disease.

A surgeon in Texas admitted that he had negligently removed a man's healthy right lung, leaving a malignant tumor in the left one. Nearly three years after the botched surgery, the sixty-two-year-old man died.

Recently, in Massachusetts, a surgeon removed a patient's healthy kidney, leaving the cancer-filled kidney intact.

In the New York area, lab results showing a pregnancy in a woman about to have a hysterectomy never reached the doctor. The woman had her uterus removed.

In Florida, a physically fit forty-four-year-old mother of three almost-grown children agreed to a vaginal hysterectomy in hopes that the procedure would relieve her painful monthly cramps. Less than two weeks later, she was dead from a massive infection. Documents filed in a subsequent civil action, later settled, claimed that the infection was introduced by a non-sterile catheter nurses had inserted into the patient's bladder.

The State Health Department of New York pointed to "serious systemic problems" at a New York hospital that led to six blood-transfusion errors in five years, one of which contributed to the death of a patient. According to the department, the errors arose because "technicians, nurses, and residents disregarded rules for insuring that the right blood reached the right patient."

In Boston, an award-winning health columnist died after a chemotherapy error. The thirty-nine-year-old writer received four times the normal dosage of a highly toxic cancer-fighting drug. Investigations revealed that a similar error had almost killed another woman two days earlier. That patient survived, but suffered severe heart damage. Similarly, in Chicago, a forty-one-year-old man being treated for testicular cancer (which currently is curable in about 95 percent of cases) died after he received a chemotherapy overdose.

In a well-known cancer center, a neurosurgical oncologist operated on the healthy right side of an Indian woman's brain, instead of another patient (male) whose name was somewhat similar and who had a brain tumor on the right side.

Libby Zion, daughter of two prominent journalists, was admitted to a major New York City teaching hospital with agitation, a high fever, and an earache. As prescribed by a first-year intern, she was given a shot of Demerol to control the agitation despite the fact that she was taking Nardil, an antidepressant. Demerol should never be given to anyone who is taking Nardil. Libby Zion died a few hours after being given the Demerol.

Unfortunately, medication errors are shockingly frequent in hospitals. A Harvard School of Public Health study of two major Boston hospitals over a six-month period found that more than 40 percent of the most serious drug reactions in hospitals, largely caused by doctors' and nurses' mistakes, may be preventable. Many of these errors were caused by one or more violations occurring in the five rules for the correct administration of medication:

- Right patient
- Right drug
- Right dose
- Right route
- Right time

That means the wrong patient may have gotten a drug correctly prescribed for someone else or the right patient may have gotten the correct medication, but the wrong dosage. Usually, these mistakes cause little harm—a rash, some nausea, or a rapid heartbeat. But in the Harvard study, of the 334 drug errors investigated, 14 were life-threatening and 30 were considered serious.

Sometimes, it isn't another patient who gets your medication and it isn't by mistake. Every physician knows of at least one doctor, nurse, or other hospital worker who is or was drug addicted. But these addictions can also be hazardous to you as a patient. Not only may your care be compromised by an addicted health professional, but you also may not receive your prescribed dosage of pain medication. Patients have been known to get only a minimal dosage of pain medicine or even simple saline when doctors, nurses, and other hospital personnel (including those with access to the pharmacy) addicted to the drug, water down the patient's medication, taking the remainder of the dosage for their own use. When the patient's physician hears that the patient is still in pain, he or she may raise the dosage, inadvertently overdosing the patient.

Learn the names of drugs being prescribed for you and always ask the nurse for the name of the drug and dosage you are being given, regardless of if it is an injection, spray, transdermal patch, IV, pill, or liquid. If it isn't what you have been told you'll be getting or the medication looks different in any way, ask the nurse to double-check. To be certain that the proper medication is being given to the correct patient, ask, "Do you know my name and what I'm being treated for?" After taking a medication, report any unusual sensations such as chills, a flushing sensation, headache, chest pain or pressure, and so on immediately.

Also tell the nurse immediately if you have swelling or redness at the site of an IV line, if you have trouble breathing or chest pain after receiving a blood transfusion, or basically, any reactions that are different or unexpected. It may be a perfectly normal side effect; if so, you should have been fully informed to expect these symptoms. Or it could be a possible allergic reaction or other sign that something is very wrong. Your immediate concern and call for help could save your life.

Sometimes, the error is the fault of the doctor who hurriedly scrawls his or her instructions on a chart or prescription pad. The jokes about doctors' penmanship ring hollow in the ears of someone who has lost a family member because the physician's illegible handwriting was misread. According to John Ruckdeschel, director of the H. Lee Moffitt Cancer Center & Research Institute in Tampa, Florida, "A spelling mistake can be a problem; a missed decimal point is lethal."

Pitfalls also occur with drugs that resemble one another or have similar packaging. Some vials resemble others in size, shape, or color, often causing fatal results. In Colorado, a veteran nurse inadvertently used *potassium* chloride (which can stop the heart) to flush a catheter, rather than 0.9 percent *sodium* chloride. The two liquids were contained in almost identical-looking bottles.

Seven cases in New York were recorded where cancer patients accidentally received 300 mg of a drug called cisplatin, rather than 300 mg of carboplatin, the correct chemotherapy. Confusion between these two drugs is, unfortunately, common, and possibly fatal. Warnings need to be placed on the drug containers and computers need to be programmed to flag mix-ups before the medication is given to unknowing cancer patients hoping to be cured or at least to have their cancer go into remission. Despite (or perhaps, due to) computers, medication errors continue to be the leading cause of accidents in hospitals. Many of them could be prevented.

Hospitals need to instill extra checks and safeguards any time medications are ordered from their pharmacy. Physicians are hardly infallible. They can err by prescribing the wrong dosages, forgetting what other medications the patient is taking or what allergies there may be. There should be verification both at the hospital pharmacy end where the prescription begins and at the nursing end *before* any drug is given to the patient.

Why is so little information reported when these and other medical errors occur? Mainly because the reporting is based primarily on an honor system. Hospitals are expected to report their own mistakes and accidents to their state authorities. They then are requested to investigate how the unfortunate event(s) happened, determine who was responsible, and declare how they will prevent similar mistakes from taking place in the future. While this procedure may sound good in theory, it is an idealistic program doomed to failure as hospital reports of errors and omissions usually reflect only the tip of the iceberg.

HOW CAN YOU PROTECT YOURSELF?

Sadly, additional anecdotes such as those above could fill the remainder of this book and probably two additional volumes. But the ones mentioned are sufficient to pose the question: How can I protect myself or a loved one from these hazards and potentially fatal errors?

Some events are just mistakes that you as the patient or family member can do nothing about, no matter how vigilant, knowledgeable, or caring you may be. Such a situation took place in Melbourne, Florida, when construction workers inadvertently cut off the oxygen supply to fifty-six hospital patients. One patient, a fifty-five-year-old woman recovering from orthopaedic surgery, went into cardiac arrest, slipped into a coma, and died four days later.

In many cases, however, family and patients can avert possible disasters by becoming informed about the illness as well as treatment procedures and medications; asking questions; and trusting their instincts. Having a family member or friend in *constant* attendance doubles your vigilance and is vitally important, especially if you are unconscious or otherwise unable to defend yourself.

Here are fourteen ways in which you can protect yourself against hospital hazards:

1. Ask those caring for you to wash their hands before touching you or permitting medical equipment to come into contact with you.

2. Know what medications you are taking, why, and what your prescribed dosage is. If a pill, capsule, or liquid looks different from what you've been taking, bring it to the nurse's attention *before* taking it. It may be that it's just the generic brand; or it may be that it's the wrong medication.

3. Know when you are supposed to get a particular medication and tell the nurse if you don't. One of the most frequent drug errors is forgetting to administer it. Nurses get busy and time slips by. On the other hand, if someone comes in with your meds, thinking that your nurse forgot to give them to you when you've already gotten them, pull out your chart and show the record of it. That's another reason why you need to know the nurses' names, so you can say who gave you the medication and when.

4. Be sure you know what is being dripped into your veins through the IV line. If you can't remember, write down the names of the medications, how often you should receive them, and what the correct dosage is. Do this even if you are only receiving saline to keep the line open.

5. Tell the nurse *immediately* if you have any unexpected reaction to a medication or an IV. This includes (but is not limited to) a pain or burning sensation, shortness of breath or trouble breathing, dizziness, confusion, tightness in your chest, numbness, or itching.

6. If your roommate or your roommate's visitors are coughing or sneezing, have skin infections, or show other overt signs of illness, ask to be reassigned to a different room. Most germs are airborne or are transmitted through direct contact, such as the toilet or sink in the bathroom, door handle, or a common chair or telephone.

7. Before beginning respiratory therapy, ask how the equipment is sterilized. The hardware should be autoclaved (heated to 212°F). The software should be disposable. Contaminated equipment can spread infection quickly into your lungs.

8. Use a permanent felt-tip marker on your skin to indicate which side of your body is the proper one for surgery. That way you can protect yourself even after you're under anesthesia. Mistakes can and do occur. You'll feel better knowing that you have added one extra precaution against errors happening to you by marking the correct spot "Cut here."

9. Know your blood type, especially if you are not having autologous transfusions. Although the chances of your receiving mismatched blood are slight (one in 600,000), such a mistake can be fatal. Unfortunately, just knowing your blood type (*e.g.*, A, B+, O-) is not sure-proof as most transfusion reactions are due to differences in one of the hundreds of minor sub-types.

10. Never eat undercooked eggs or any hospital food that smells or looks "funny," is not on your specific diet list, or contains (or may contain) anything to which you have allergic reactions. If you are inadvertently given a food tray before you are due to undergo surgery, don't eat it.

11. To serve as a reminder for nurses, aides, and physicians, make a sign from poster board listing your name, room number, serious allergies, and chronic medical conditions and tape it over the head of your bed. This display can help alleviate errors made by staff who may be fatigued, frustrated, under stress or time constraints, or otherwise preoccupied.

    (Some hospitals even furnish bulletin boards over the head of patients' beds for this specific purpose. If yours doesn't, suggest it.)

12. If you have a question, ask it, even if the doctor or nurse is edging out the door. There is no such thing

as a "stupid" question. It is your right as a patient to have your questions answered.

13. If there is another patient on the floor with the same or similar name to yours, ask your doctor to change your floor.

14. If you feel that a mistake is being made, always speak up. Trust your instincts. Be assertive. If you're wrong, you're wrong, but you'll still be alive.

Safety and Security: Infant Abductions, Rapes, Violence, Falls, Fires, and Other Dangers

Most people's perception of a hospital is that it's a safe place where you are free from harm, can relax your guard knowing that you are being cared for (the "spa" or "nursery" image), and can expect an unhurried professional staff to work in harmony to make you well again. Unfortunately, that is not the reality.

In their winter 1995–96 issue, *The Journal of Healthcare Protection Management* published the results of the 1994 security survey conducted by the International Association for Healthcare Security and Safety (IAHSS), a non-profit organization of professional health-care security and safety executives worldwide. Two hundred and eighty hospitals in the United States and Canada (representing forty-three states and four Canadian provinces) participated in this survey, including those located in urban-suburban, rural, and inner-city areas. The bed sizes of these hospitals ranged from the smallest (1–100 beds) to those with over 1,000 beds.

The results of that survey showed that in 1994, 20,254 crimes occurred on the premises of the reporting hospitals. They included

30 homicides, 25 suicides, 1,577 assaults—including 9 rapes and 65 other sexual assaults, 193 robberies, with 60 of them armed robberies, 941 burglaries, 973 auto thefts, 42 arsons, 14,967 larcenies, 3,124 incidents of vandalism, and 115 incidents of fraud. (The category of infant kidnappings was eliminated for 1994 and the figures included in other areas.) So much for a safe haven.

According to Bonnie Michelman, Director of Police and Security at Boston's Massachusetts General and president of the IAHSS, "Hospitals are a microcosm of society. There is a joint responsibility required of both staff and patients and their families. Hospitals dance a delicate line. They must protect their patients and staff while at the same time, they can't feel like Fort Knox. We're not a health fair. We can't lock our doors at 5:00 P.M."

This Scylla and Charybdis of a dilemma often creates hard feelings and frustration from those requiring legitimate access to the hospital as well as posing real danger to those within the institution—patients, visitors, and staff alike. Most hospitals, because of their size and complexities as well as today's financial constraints, have become impersonal and overwhelming medical mazes. As patients are shuttled along the conveyor belt of care, they are seen by a myriad of staff, usually a minimum of fifteen to twenty different people, few of whom will have the opportunity to get to know them as individuals. For most of the personnel, patients are nameless faces—a product just passing through the system.

Ask an X-ray technician or phlebotomist (the person who draws your blood) to describe and name the last patient he or she saw; few can. Ask the same question to a member of the housekeeping staff who just cleaned a patient's room, the transporter who pushed a frightened patient on a gurney to the holding area outside of the operating room, or the attendant who just delivered a food tray (perhaps just out of the patient's reach), and most likely you'll get a blank look.

Many hospitals decry this impersonal approach and have mission statements that avow they will try (and most do try) to individualize and humanize each patient. But the truth is that in today's world of medicine, in which insurance company dictates pressure hospitals to reduce length of stays to "drive by and we'll heal you" duration and continue to contain costs by cutting full-time employees, it is a difficult, if not impossible, task.

Hospitals, even small community and rural facilities, have become too large with too many people wandering about to keep track of all the players. It's hard to know who's staff, consultant, volunteer, or salesperson; to distinguish a patient from a family member, or a visitor from a volunteer; or to keep track of the ever-present contractors and laborers, those delivering flowers and newspapers, service people repairing patients' TV sets, and members of the clergy. Ultimately, this combination of a strolling cast of characters along with cutbacks in staff that bring in a revolving door of faceless part-time workers to supplement full-time employees, leaves the door wide open to many of the hospital hazards, such as nosocomial infections, drug and surgical errors, infant abductions, patient attacks and rapes, falls, violence, thefts, and other dangers.

INFANT ABDUCTIONS

Although infant abductions are not the most common threat to safety and security in the hospital, they are the most publicized by the media, probably because of their emotional appeal. From 1983 to 1996, eighty-nine babies from birth to six months of age were abducted from U.S. hospitals. While this number may not seem large, it is eighty-nine too many for the families involved. According to the security director of one major hospital, the problem becomes worse in hospitals with rooming-in facilities (most of them today), which allow the infant to sleep in the same room with the mother rather than in the traditional nursery. When mom's asleep or in the bathroom, someone can creep in and steal the baby. Statistics from the National Center for Missing & Exploited Children reveal that 56 percent of infants abducted from health-care facilities are taken from the mother's room, with 76 percent of those occurring between the hours of 6:00 A.M. and 6:00 P.M.

Older hospitals tend to have more abductions than the newer ones, says a security officer from a major southern hospital, because they have too many exterior access doors, leaving security gaps.

The "typical" baby thief is a woman from fourteen to forty-five and usually in her early thirties. She probably does not have a criminal record. She either cannot have children or has lost her own child. She may feel under pressure to have a baby in order to keep a boyfriend or husband. She spends time in the hospital, observing what the staff at that particular hospital wears, then goes to a uniform shop and buys identical scrubs or uniform. She also may steal them from an unlocked supply closet or locker room at the hospital itself.

According to a report created by the National Center for Missing & Exploited Children, "The vast majority of these women take on the 'role' of a nurse and represent themselves as such to the victim mother and anyone else in the room with the mother." The fake nurse then claims she needs to take the baby to be weighed or photographed and leaves with the infant, often exiting hurriedly through a back stairwell.

It is not unusual for hospital administrators who are concerned about infant safety and other security actions to hire security and safety consultants to move freely about their facility, checking the effectiveness of security measures. Bonnie Michelman tells of such an assignment in her role as president of the IAHSS.

"I was asked to check out the security for newborns in a particular hospital," she said. "Wearing a professional-looking business suit, I walked into the hospital and took the elevator to the maternity floor. No one asked for identification or said a thing when I walked down the hall, entered the newborn nursery, and picked up one of the infants. Nor did anyone stop me when I took that baby out of the nursery, back into the elevator, and down to the lobby. I walked out of the hospital and put the baby in the astonished (and chagrined) CEO's arms. 'I think you need to improve your newborn security,' I told him."

What can you do to prevent your baby from being abducted from the hospital?

The National Center for Missing & Exploited Children offers these guidelines:[1]

1. At some point *before* the birth of your baby, investigate security procedures at the facility where you plan to give birth to your baby and request a copy of the facility's written guidelines on procedures for "special care" and security procedures in the maternity ward. Make sure you know all of the facility's procedures that are in place to safeguard your infant while staying in that facility.

2. While it is normal for new parents to be anxious, being deliberately watchful over the newborn infant is of paramount importance.

3. Never leave your infant out of your direct line-of-sight—even when you go to the bathroom or take a nap. If you leave the room or plan to go to sleep, alert the nurses to take the infant back to the nursery or have a family member watch the baby.

4. After admission to the facility, ask about hospital protocols concerning the routine nursery procedures, feeding and visitation hours, and security measures.

5. Do not give your infant to *anyone* without properly verified hospital identification. Find out what additional or special identification is being worn to further

---

1 *"What Parents Need to Know" is from* Healthcare Professionals: Guidelines on Prevention and Response to Infant Abductions *by John B. Rabun, Jr., ACSW, and reprinted with permission of the National Center for Missing & Exploited Children (NCMEC). Copyright © NCMEC 1989, 1991, 1992, 1993, and 1996. All rights reserved.*

identify those hospital personnel who have authority to handle the infant.

6. Become familiar with the hospital staff who work in the maternity unit. During short stays in the hospital, be sure you know the nurse assigned to you and your infant.

7. Question unfamiliar persons entering your room or inquiring about your infant—even if they are in hospital attire or seem to have a reason for being there. Alert the nurses' station immediately.

8. Determine where your infant will be when taken for tests, and how long the tests will take. Find out who has authorized the tests. If you are uncomfortable with anyone who requests to take your baby or is unable to clarify what testing is being done or why your baby is being taken from your room, it is appropriate to go with your baby to observe the procedure.

9. For your records to take home, have at least one color photograph of your infant taken (full, front-face view) and compile a complete written description of your infant, including hair and eye color, length, weight, date of birth, and specific physical attributes.

10. At some point *after* the birth of your baby, but *before* discharge from the facility, request a set of written guidelines on the procedures for any follow-up care extended by the facility that will be scheduled to take place in your home. Do not allow anyone into your home who claims to be affiliated with the facility without properly verified hospital identification. Find out what additional or special identification is being worn to further identify those staff members who have authority to enter your home.

11. Consider the risk you may be taking when permitting your infant's birth announcement to be published in the newspaper. Birth announcements should never include the family's home address and should be limited to the parents' surname(s).

12. The use of outdoor decorations to announce the infant's arrival, such as mylar balloons, large floral wreaths, wooden storks, and other lawn ornaments, is not recommended.

13. Only allow persons into your home who are well-known by the mother. It is ill-advised to allow anyone into your home who is a mere acquaintance, especially if met briefly since you became pregnant or gave birth to your baby. There have been several cases in which an abductor has made initial contact with a mother and baby in the hospital setting and then subsequently abducted the infant at the family home. If anyone should arrive at the home claiming to be affiliated with the health-care facility where the infant was born, remember to follow the procedures outlined in number 10.

    In addition, there have been cases in which initial contact with a mother and baby was made in other settings such as shopping malls. Family members should exercise a high degree of diligence when home with the baby.

After having a baby, it's normal to experience a flood of emotions—including fatigue, excitement, anxiety, and nervousness. But don't let your guard down. Remember that newborns usually are not physically carried in a nurse's arms, but are transported in wheeled bassinets. Be alert and report any suspected infant abduction to the nurses' station immediately.

Don't be timid about questioning your proposed maternity facility *before* your due date. Ask if the hospital you plan to use has security closed-circuit television that is properly monitored and has cameras that are in working order. Do they use infant bracelet alarms and access control? What type of identification is used for those with clearance to handle the babies? Has the staff received training annually on how to prevent infant abduction?

"Become knowledgeable," Ms. Michelman suggests. "Check the crime rate for the hospital you are considering. Learn what security measures they have in place for obstetrics." Enjoy your new baby, but stay alert.

PATIENT ATTACKS AND RAPES

According to the 1994 survey by the IAHSS, "The second most common area of criminal activity was in patient rooms. [Note:The most common area was at employee work stations.] Thefts, assaults, and disorderly conduct were the most numerous types of crime to occur in patient rooms." Also revealed in this same survey was that the top three categories of perpetrators of most hospital crime are visitors, patients, and hospital employees, although as most hospital crime goes unsolved, it is hard to provide an accurate accounting of who is committing them. Other categories of perpetrators of crime include physicians, vendors, and "other."

With chilling frequency the media expose cases of hospital attacks or rape—comatose women impregnated, women in surgical recovery units awakening from anesthetic-imposed sleep to discover they are being sexually abused, or confused elderly female patients with bleeding and lacerated genitals, unable to explain who took advantage of them.

A woman hospitalized and recovering from the effects of a recluse spider bite awoke to find a patient from the psychiatric floor standing over her, beating on her, and ripping off the bed clothes. The woman, attached to an IV line, struggled to find the nurse call button, only to realize it had fallen off the bed and was dangling beyond her reach. Fortunately, the floor nurse overheard her cries and was able to distract the psychiatric patient and escort her out of the woman's room.

Although the security obviously was lax on the psychiatric floor in this case, the woman also could have been rescued more promptly if the call button had been secured to the sheets by her hand or attached to the bed railing in a convenient location.

Before going to sleep in a hospital, always check to be sure there's a light in the bathroom and that the nurse call button is close at hand. While the emergency may not be an attack by another patient (or member of the hospital staff or visitor), you could need immediate help for bleeding, chest pains, or other distress situations.

In Connecticut, a paralyzed, mute woman suffering from Lou Gehrig's Disease claimed that she was sexually assaulted in her hospital bed two days in a row by a male respiratory therapist. According to reports by the Associated Press, the man would close the curtains around her bed between 8:00 A.M. and 10:00 A.M. and touch her as she lay awake. Because of her illness, she was unable to scream or move. Her husband realized something was wrong when he visited her and saw tears rolling down her cheeks. Using an alphabet board, the woman was able to blink at letters to spell out a description of her assailant to the police. Later, she identified the hospital worker to police by blinking "yes" at his picture.

While the alleged sexual attack on this woman, as well as the woman who was attacked by the psychiatric patient, could have been prevented if someone had been with the patient at all times, this often is not possible, especially in long-term situations.

Many hospitals now require that a minimum of two nurses staff recovery rooms and other areas where unconscious or helpless patients may be vulnerable to attack. Ask what security measures are in place at your hospital.

Patients are extremely vulnerable to an assault within a hospital setting. They are the perfect victims—available (the bedroom door is never locked) and defenseless. Some are even physically restrained, because of their illness, by a cast, a catheter, or an IV. Although patients are advised not to bring valuables into the hospital, many disregard the warning and are robbed of cash, jewelry, purses, valuable picture frames, laptop computers, and radios, sometimes even in broad daylight as the patient sleeps or worse, watches helplessly.

Visitors in the hospital parking lot or parking garage are also at risk. A robber may loiter, watching for a potential victim— someone well-dressed, wearing expensive jewelry, and one who seems distracted by grief, fatigue, stress, or concern. Remind family members and friends who visit you in the hospital to remain alert as they head for the parking garage or parking lot. If they feel uneasy in any way, they should ask a hospital security guard to escort them to their car. Many hospitals now monitor their parking areas with security patrols and closed-circuit television.

Don't relax your guard and be lulled into false security because you think any area of the hospital (parking garage, hallway, elevator, and so on) is being monitored by closed-circuit television, however. The system may not be monitored continually, a camera may be out of order, or some of the cameras may be "dummies," that is, fake cameras used to supplement the real equipment. Stay alert.

VIOLENCE

The threat of violence is seldom discussed or even thought about by most patients in a hospital, yet it, too, is very real. According to the 1994 IAHSS crime survey, although inner-city hospitals made up only 33.9 percent of the hospitals completing the survey, 45.6 percent of health-care crime occurred there, with 67.6 percent of the reported crime-related, health-care injuries. Yet violence occurs in private hospitals, "boutique" hospitals, community hospitals, and surprisingly, even in rural hospitals as well. In fact, the same 1994 survey revealed that urban-suburban locations had the fastest-growing crime rate.

Not all of the violence stems from drug usage or gang activity. Domestic violence is a major contributor. Once a victim of domestic abuse is hospitalized, the abuser's anger and frustration may be accentuated by guilt and embarrassment, and violence can erupt within the hospital room itself.

More than half of all reported acts of violence in a hospital take place in the emergency department. Many of those in emergency rooms are carrying guns or other weapons. Fear, resentment at having to wait, intoxication or drug use, domestic disputes, and continuation of gang wars all may be acted out in this crowded playing field. Emergency department physicians estimate that more than 75 percent of patients and visitors to some inner-city emergency departments are under the influence of drugs.[2]

While the public may be unaware of some of these dangers, the hospital administrations are not. A large part of any hospital budget today is spent on safety and security measures. While often not publicized, many hospitals have created entire professional security departments. The security force is charged with providing greater safety measures to protect patients, staff, and visitors. But they cannot do it alone. Everyone—patients and visitors alike—must remain active and aware in the hospital setting and be ready to report any suspicious situation to the proper hospital authorities.

What can you do if you suspect violence is about to break out—or are caught in a verbal or physical crossfire? Mark A. Hart, assistant security director at Southwest Texas Methodist Hospital in San Antonio, has these suggestions:

1. Don't get involved in a conversation with someone who seems about to lose control; instead, quietly go to the desk or security guard and report the information to the professional.

---

[2]*Russell L. Collins,* Hospital Security *(Stoneham, MA: Butterworth-Heinemann, 1992), 286.*

2. Don't stare or glare at anyone talking or complaining loudly or who appears tense and angry; it could be taken as a confrontational act.

3. If violence breaks out, don't try to be a hero. Never attempt to subdue the person yourself.

FALLS

Patient falls are a major concern for hospitals. It isn't just the elderly who fall. Patients of all ages, weak from illness or surgery, dizzy from side effects of multiple medications, or fatigued from too much time in bed, often fall as they try to get to the bathroom. Some fall trying to climb over the bed rails, which were put up to *prevent* their falling out of bed. Many patients get up during the night to go to the bathroom, forget that they are tethered to an IV line or catheter, and trip, which may cause painful rips in delicate tissue along with possible hip fractures, fractures in other areas, concussions, and soft-tissue injuries from the fall.

Staff negligence also can be responsible for a patient's falling. An eighty-four-year-old male cancer patient, in complete control of his mental faculties, was brought down from his room for a bone scan. For previous scans, one of his adult children had remained with him in the room during this tedious but non-invasive procedure. This time, however, the technician insisted that his daughter wait in the waiting room. "It's too crowded in here," he told her.

With some reluctance, the woman kissed her father good-bye and left to find the waiting room. An hour later, the technician came in and told her the procedure was complete and that her father would be returned to his room. She thanked him and then, almost as an afterthought, said, "Who is with my father now?"

"Now?" repeated the technician. "No one. I just called the orderly."

Shoving the technician aside, the woman flew into the bone-scan room. Her father lay crumpled on the floor, his gown wadded up over his hips. A trickle of blood oozed from his forehead and he was moaning from the pain caused by a now-shattered hip bone. Unattended, he had rolled off the narrow table used for the scan and had fallen to the floor below. Although his cancer remained in remission, his hip failed to heal properly. He remained bedridden for four months, when he died from complications of pneumonia.

Here are fifteen ways to help prevent hospital falls:

1. Keep your eyeglasses in reach on the nightstand and put them on before getting up. Visual acuity may be affected by fever, residual effects of anesthesia, or medications.

2. Make sure the bed is cranked down to its normal low position before trying to get out of bed.

3. If the side rails are up (they may be if you are heavily medicated, feverish, or recovering from the effects of anesthesia), do *not* try to climb over them. Ring for a nurse to put them down.

4. Move the bedside table away from the bed before going to sleep at night so you don't trip over it.

5. Dangle your feet over the side of the bed for a few minutes to regain your balance before getting out of bed.

6. To prevent slipping, wear slippers with rubberized soles that won't flop off your feet.

7. Wait for the nurse or an aide to answer your call button if you feel the least bit shaky or dizzy.

8. Ask the nurse for a night-light in the bathroom.

9. Take care that the sash from your bathrobe hasn't slipped down, which could cause you to trip.

10. Use your walker as directed.

11. Watch for wet floors; they may be as slippery as ice.

12. Move slowly, especially if you've been feverish or bedridden for a while. Even astronauts lose muscle tone when they've been in weightlessness for a period of time.

13. Be sure that dresser drawers and closet doors are shut before going to bed so you won't bang into them in the dark.

14. Ask your last visitor or the nurse to move the chairs in order to clear the path from the bed to the bathroom, in case you have to get up at night.

15. If you're a caregiver, not the patient, remain with your loved one for scans and other procedures unless you can be assured that he or she will be constantly monitored by someone in the room.

FIRES

Numerous studies reveal that 10 percent of health-care facilities have had some type of fire break out during their existence. (Note: Nursing home facilities as well as hospitals were included in this research.) According to security officers interviewed for this book, one of the major causes is careless smoking, even in areas where smoking is prohibited. Hospital fires can be especially deadly because many of the patients, such as the pediatric population, the elderly, those heavily medicated, the mentally or physically handicapped, and the extremely ill, are unable to evacuate the premises on their own. Because they are ill or recovering from surgery, even

---

☞ Remember these lifesaving tips listed below; patients (and their visitors) have a responsibility to help prevent fires. Follow your hospital's regulations concerning smoking.

- *Never sneak a smoke if smoking is prohibited; especially never smoke in your bed or when oxygen is in use.*

- *If there is a designated smoking area, always snuff your cigarette out in the specially provided receptacle or flush it down the toilet. Don't put it out in a paper or Styrofoam cup filled with water as the water can be absorbed by the filters in several butts and the cup can then catch on fire.*

- *Never drop your cigarette in the wastebasket.*

- *Be alert for others (patients or visitors) who disregard the hospital's smoking rules and report them to a security officer or a member of the nursing staff.*

- *Do not use any electrical equipment, such as a radio, tape recorder, computer, and so on, without clearing it with the nurse or engineering staff.*

- *Call a nurse immediately if you smell smoke; if no one answers your call button, notify the hospital switchboard.*

---

ambulatory patients may panic at the first mention of fire and be less likely to follow instructions pertaining to their safety.

Knowing this, most hospitals give all employees annual training in how to respond to a fire. According to an article by Douglas A. Campbell, director of safety, security, and risk management at Robert Wood Johnson University Hospital in New Brunswick, New Jersey, most hospitals use a fire response system called RACE. The acronym represents the various steps the hospital staff follows in case of a fire. They include:

- Removing people from danger
- Activating a fire alarm
- Closing doors and windows
- Extinguishing fire and escaping

As you can see, the first step always is to remove patients from danger. If fire should break out in the hospital while you're a patient there, don't panic. Frightened patients can get in the way of the fire brigade, undermining their ability to function properly. If you're ambulatory, calmly follow the directions given to you by the medical staff. If you're bedridden, someone will be assigned to see to your well-being. Hospital staffs are trained in evacuation procedures in case of fire or other disasters; the plan usually breaks down only if someone (most often, a patient) panics.

Cooperate with the trained hospital staff. They'll get you out safely.

DANGEROUS DINING

Although many patients look forward to mealtime to relieve the boredom of hospital routine, those food trays may be serving up lethal lunches and potentially disastrous dinners.

Food Allergies

Food allergies you had at home don't suddenly disappear in the hospital. Yet many patients never see (or ask to see) the hospital's dietitian. Those coming in through the emergency department are often too distraught to remember to tell anyone that their throat closes up when they eat fish—or that their heart beats erratically if they eat anything with peanuts or peanut oil.

Always check the name on your food tray to be sure that your food tray hasn't been mixed up with that of your roommate or next-door neighbor.

Drug Interactions with Certain Food

If you're hospitalized, chances are good that you're taking more medications than you were at home. Often it's as many as nine different drugs at once. While these medications are (or should be) listed on your chart, their combined effect together or with food may be overlooked.

Certain drugs, such as Pen G penicillins and tetracyclines, lose their effectiveness if taken orally right after eating certain foods. Whenever you're brought medication, always tell your nurse that you've just eaten, regardless if it's a snack brought to you from a visitor or your hospital meal.

Other drugs, such as the antidepressants known as the monoamine oxidase inhibitors (MAOs)—which includes Parnate, Nardil, and Marplan—can trigger dangerously high blood pressure when taken with a number of foods, including (but not limited to) aged cheese, Chianti wine, beer, yogurt, chicken liver, chocolate, bananas, soy sauce, bologna, salami, and avocado.

Recent studies question the wisdom of taking medications with grapefruit juice—especially with blood-pressure medications and antihistamines. There are ingredients called flavonoids in grapefruit juice that seem to intensify the levels of these and other drugs. In some cases, toxicity may result. To be safe, wait at least four hours after taking medicine to drink grapefruit juice.

Even a sweet treat like licorice, brought to you by a well-meaning visitor, can be dangerous and potentially fatal, as copious amounts of licorice can draw potassium from your system and dangerously interact with medications such as Lanoxin, which is used for congestive heart failure and disturbances of the heart rhythm. Before you ingest any food (including seemingly harmless treats such as candy or gum), check with your physician.

It's important for you to know what medications you're taking as well as their potential side effects. Few people will experience *all* side effects listed for a medication, but you should be aware of what they could be. Your chart may say that you're not to eat specific foods because of the particular drugs you're getting, but if your tray is mixed up with your roommate's or that of the patient next door, the food you eat could be lethal.

An excellent book on the subject of medicine and food interactions as well as the effects of drugs on other drugs is *The Consumer's Guide to Drug Interactions.* While it doesn't list all of the possible dangerous interactions, it makes us more aware that food can have an effect on the medications we take and to report any symptoms experienced to the charge nurse immediately.

Food Poisoning

Hospitals, like other large institutions, prepare food in massive amounts with ample opportunity for improper handling. Food may be kept warm on steam heating units until being transported to the patients' rooms or may sit on trays in hallways for long periods of time waiting to be delivered by understaffed aides. Either situation provides an ideal atmosphere for bacteria to grow. Food handlers may cough or sneeze, contaminating utensils or the food itself.

While ordinarily the amount of contamination or bacteria in food may not be harmful to a healthy person, it can have serious effects on critically ill patients, those with liver disease, infants and small children, or those with a compromised immune system. Dehydration (from vomiting) could become a problem, especially in infants and elderly patients.

Never eat any food that smells, tastes, or looks "funny." Report any nausea, vomiting, diarrhea, or abdominal cramping that develops one to six hours after eating to your nurse.

Choking

Choking can be a potential problem at mealtime. Be sure you're sitting upright, not just propped up on your pillow. If you can't crank the bed up yourself, ring for someone to do it for you. Cut your food into small pieces and take little bites. If you've recently had an anesthetic or are on pain medications, be especially careful as the drugs used also affect the part of the brain that controls swallowing.

Cut your food into smaller pieces than you would normally and consciously chew it before swallowing. Never gulp your food down. You might as well be leisurely about your dining; you've got no place else to go. Patients with dentures, those on pain medication, and elderly patients may especially have trouble chewing or swallowing because of the effects of the various drugs they're taking. (If you wear dentures and remove them while eating, always put them in the designated container provided. Patients often leave their dentures on the food tray or in a napkin and the dentures accidentally get thrown out.)

If you are a caregiver to a patient and you can't remain with him or her all of the time, at least try to arrange to be there or have a substitute caregiver there during mealtimes. It can be a potentially dangerous time. Patients are vulnerable then as they are alone and propped up away from the call button. With the noise and commotion of meals being delivered, they probably could not be heard if they were to call out. If they were to choke on food due to weakness, after effects of the anesthesia, or side effects of their medications, no one would hear.

Unreachable Food

Often hospitalized patients don't eat well, not because the food is inedible (which it also may be), but because they can't reach it. Food servers pop into a room, put the tray down on the table, and exit to hurry into the next room, without checking to see if the patient can even reach the food. It isn't only the elderly who may have difficulty sitting up and getting to the food; those who have had breast, abdominal, or chest surgery also may not be able to fend for themselves.

If you can't be with your family member throughout the day, ask when trays are delivered (don't expect them at the normal times) and be there during mealtime or arrange for someone else to be. Eating can present many challenges when you're ill—just taking a straw out of its wrapper, removing the cardboard cover on the coffee container, or lifting the cover off the plate itself may seem overwhelming. A patient may just be too tired or weak to cut up meat or even to open the packet of silverware. Many patients just don't bother. When the food server comes to remove the tray, they usually don't take time to ask why nothing was eaten. So the patient becomes weaker, not from the illness, but the lack of proper nourishment.

If you're the patient, ask the food server to move the tray within reach or ring for help, that is, of course, if you can reach your call button.

Intravenous Feeding and Tube Feeding

Although not the most satisfying way to enjoy a meal, IV feeding does provide nourishment for those unable or unwilling to eat. With IV feedings, nutrients are put into a catheter (tubing) that goes into a large central vein; with tube feedings, the tubing is inserted through the nose and into the stomach or small intestine. With both, there is some danger of infection. Tell the nurse immediately if you develop swelling, redness, or pain in your arms, hands, legs, feet, or at the site of the catheter.

You also could experience some nausea, vomiting, stomach pain, or diarrhea. Don't suffer in silence. Call the nurse immediately if any of these symptoms arise. He or she can make changes that can make you more comfortable.

Non Per Os (NPO)

"*Non per os*" is Latin for "nothing by mouth." It usually is written on a card tacked over your bed the evening before you're to undergo surgery, because you could vomit the contents in your stomach under anesthetic and aspirate the matter into your lungs.

Nevertheless, as human error can always raise its ugly head, avoid eating anything after you are NPO *even* if it's brought into your room, is placed on your tray table, and has your name on it.

Packages from Home

Never bring your own medications into the hospital or take anything, even a so-called "simple" aspirin from home, without your physician's expressed permission. Your doctor will usually order your former medications from the hospital pharmacy if he or she feels you should continue to take them. It's vital for the health-care professionals to know exactly what you are ingesting. Otherwise, they may inadvertently give you a medication that could have dangerous, if not fatal, side effects when it interacts with what you took from home. Never bring illegal drugs or alcohol to the hospital either.

As you can see, your safety and security within the hospital setting depends upon many varying factors. But you cannot rely strictly on the hospital administration and medical staff to make safety and security as near perfect as is humanly possible. You and your family and friends must become non-official security officers, remaining ever vigilant for situations ready to erupt.

Check on the security precautions at whatever hospital you decide to use. Ask for a tour by one of their security officers; notice the locations of security cameras, uniformed officers, and identification tags worn by staff members. Follow the suggestions listed throughout this chapter. You'll enjoy a faster recovery being alert, but not worried, about your safety while you're a patient.

CHAPTER 6

Patients' Rights

Many patients claim they know the exact moment when they begin to feel a sense of passivity and complete helplessness overtake them in the hospital. It's when they remove their clothing and replace it with a flimsy gown that barely covers their backside.

This transformation must be akin to the feeling new military recruits experience when their heads are shaved bald. In both cases it's a visible sign that you—patient or recruit—are different from the rest of the group: weaker, in need of being told what to do, and controlled by those who are wiser.

This reversion to a child-like state, however, can be extremely hazardous to your health. You cannot blindly accept what is being done to you in a hospital without question. Mistakes occur through human error. Your input, asserting your position as an active and vital part of your own health team, can help to reduce mistakes that can cause you additional expense, unnecessary exposure to pain and procedures, deformities, and sometimes even death. Assume the responsibility and stand up for yourself (even if you are lying in an uncomfortable hospital bed). If you are unable to do so, be sure there is a family member or close friend who will look out for you.

WHAT ARE A PATIENT'S RIGHTS?

In 1973, the American Hospital Association (AHA) created a list of rights for patients. It was carefully revised in 1992. While it's usually included in the packet given to new patients upon admission to the hospital, most of us don't bother to read it then because we're anxious about being hospitalized. But don't skip over this section now. It is important to read this material and understand your rights and your obligations as a patient in a hospital. You are a vital link in the health-care team; take this responsibility seriously.

A PATIENT'S BILL OF RIGHTS[1]

Introduction

Effective health care requires collaboration between patients and physicians and other health care professionals. Open and honest communication, respect for personal and professional values, and sensitivity to differences are integral to optimal patient care. As the setting for the provision of health services, hospitals must provide a foundation for understanding and respecting the rights and responsibilities of patients, their families, physicians, and other caregivers. Hospitals must ensure a health care ethic that respects the role of patients in decision making about treatment choices and other aspects of their care. Hospitals must be sensitive to cultural, racial, linguistic, religious, age, gender, and other differences as well as the needs of persons with disabilities.

The American Hospital Association presents "A Patient's Bill of Rights" with the expectation that it will contribute to more effective patient care and be supported by the hospital on behalf of the institution, its medical staff, employees, and patients. The American Hospital Association encourages health care institutions to tailor this bill of rights to their patient community by translating and/or simplifying the language of this bill of rights as may be necessary

---

[1] *The American Hospital Association's Patient's Bill of Rights. Reprinted with permission of the American Hospital Association, copyright 1992.*

to ensure that patients and their families understand their rights and responsibilities.

Bill of Rights*

1. The patient has the right to considerate and respectful care.

2. The patient has the right to and is encouraged to obtain from physicians and other direct caregivers relevant, current, and understandable information concerning diagnosis, treatment, and prognosis.

    Except in emergencies when the patient lacks decision-making capacity and the need for treatment is urgent, the patient is entitled to the opportunity to discuss and request information related to the specific procedures and/or treatment, the risks involved, the possible length of recuperation, and the medically reasonable alternatives and their accompanying risks and benefits.

    Patients have the right to know the identity of physicians, nurses, and others involved in their care, as well as when those involved are students, residents, or other trainees. The patient also has the right to know the immediate and long-term financial implications of treatment choices, insofar as they are known.

3. The patient has the right to make decisions about the plan or care prior to and during the course of treatment and to refuse a recommended treatment or plan of care to the extent permitted by law and hospital

---

*These rights can be exercised on the patient's behalf by a designated surrogate or proxy decision maker if the patient lacks decision-making capacity, is legally incompetent, or is a minor.

policy and to be informed of the medical conse-
quences of this action. In case of such refusal, the
patient is entitled to other appropriate care and services
that the hospital provides or transfer to another hospital. The hospital should notify patients of any policy
that might affect patient choice within the institution.

4. The patient has the right to have an advance directive
(such as a living will, health care proxy, or durable
power of attorney for health care) concerning treatment or designating a surrogate decision maker with
the expectation that the hospital will honor the intent
of that directive to the extent permitted by law and
hospital policy.

Health care institutions must advise patients of their
rights under state law and hospital policy to make
informed medical choices, ask if the patient has an
advance directive, and include that information in
patient records. The patient has the right to timely
information about hospital policy that may limit its
ability to implement fully a legally valid directive.

5. The patient has the right to every consideration of
privacy. Case discussion, consultation, examination, and
treatment should be conducted so as to protect each
patient's privacy.

6. The patient has the right to expect that all communications and records pertaining to his/her care will be
treated as confidential by the hospital, except in cases
as suspected abuse and public health hazards when
reporting is permitted or required by law. The patient
has the right to expect that the hospital will emphasize

the confidentiality of this information when it releases it to any other parties entitled to review information in these records.

7. The patient has the right to review the records pertaining to his/her medical care and to have the information explained or interpreted as necessary, except when restricted by law.

8. The patient has the right to expect that, within its capacity and policies, a hospital will make reasonable response to the request of a patient for appropriate and medically indicated care and services. The hospital must provide evaluation, service, and/or referral as indicated by the urgency of the case. When medically appropriate and legally permissible, or when a patient has so requested, a patient may be transferred to another facility. The institution to which the patient is to be transferred must first have accepted the patient for transfer. The patient must also have the benefit of complete information and explanation concerning the need for, risks, benefits, and alternatives to such a transfer.

9. The patient has the right to ask and be informed of the existence of business relationships among the hospital, educational institutions, other health care providers, or payers that may influence the patient's treatment and care.

10. The patient has the right to consent to or decline to participate in proposed research studies or human experimentation affecting care and treatment or requiring direct patient involvement, and to have those

studies fully explained prior to consent. A patient who declines to participate in research or experimentation is entitled to the most effective care that the hospital can otherwise provide.

11. The patient has the right to expect reasonable continuity of care when appropriate and to be informed by physicians and other caregivers of available and realistic patient care options when hospital care is no longer appropriate.

12. The patient has the right to be informed of hospital policies and practices that relate to patient care, treatment, and responsibilities. The patient has the right to be informed of available resources for resolving disputes, grievances, and conflicts, such as ethics committees, patient representatives, or other mechanisms available in the institution. The patient has the right to be informed of the hospital's charges for services and available payment methods.

The collaborative nature of health care requires that patients, or their families/surrogates, participate in their care. The effectiveness of care and patient satisfaction with the course of treatment depend, in part, on the patient fulfilling certain responsibilities. Patients are responsible for providing information about past illnesses, hospitalizations, medications, and other matters related to health status. To participate effectively in decision making, patients must be encouraged to take responsibility for requesting additional information or clarification about their health status or treatment when they do not fully understand information and instruction. Patients are also responsible for ensuring that the health care institution has a copy of their written advance directive if they have one. Patients are responsible for informing their physicians and other caregivers if they anticipate problems following prescribed treatment.

Patients should also be aware of the hospital's obligation to be reasonably efficient and equitable in providing care to other patients and the community. The hospital's rules and regulations are designed to help the hospital meet this obligation. Patients and their families are responsible for making reasonable accommodations to the needs of the hospital, other patients, medical staff, and hospital employees. Patients are responsible for providing necessary information for insurance claims and for working with the hospital to make payment arrangements, when necessary.

A person's health depends on much more than health care services. Patients are responsible for recognizing the impact of their life-style on their personal health.

Conclusion

Hospitals have many functions to perform, including the enhancement of health status, health promotion, and the prevention and treatment of injury and disease; the immediate and ongoing care and rehabilitation of patients; the education of health professionals, patients, and the community; and research. All these activities must be conducted with an overriding concern for the values and dignity of patients.

Of course, no catalog of rights can guarantee the kind of treatment patients have the right to expect, or most importantly, dictate the recognition of one's dignity as a human being. That's why you must become an informed consumer. Know your rights as a patient; be assertive. As Hillel wrote, "If I am not for myself, who will be for me? . . . If not now, when?"

HOW TO PROTECT THE CONFIDENTIALITY OF MEDICAL RECORDS AND DOCTOR/PATIENT CONVERSATIONS

"Once upon a time" it was probably true that confidentiality was the rule with patients' medical records and doctor-patient conversations. No one looked at a patient's medical chart hidden in the dented file cabinet but the trusted office secretary who had been with the doctor for at least twenty years and would have remained silent about the contents even if tortured on the rack. Doctors kept their patients' secrets even from their spouses, despite the fact that the patient and doctor's spouse were closest friends. Ah, for the good old days.

The reality of managed care and computers has made this idea a fairy tale. Contrary to what most of us assume to be so, at this writing there is no federal law protecting the privacy of medical records. Only a few states have such laws.

As more hospitals, health-care organizations, and physicians computerize their patient records, more unauthorized people will gain access to information concerning our personal lives. According to the *Harvard Health Letter,* a 1993 Louis Harris poll found that more than 25 percent of people believed their own medical information had been improperly disclosed and 34 percent of health-care professionals surveyed said records are given to unauthorized people "somewhat often."[2] What's more, this confidential information about the state of our physical and emotional health and our lifestyle can be passed along via a modem and a few key strokes to insurance and drug companies, medical equipment firms, researchers, employers and potential employers, political enemies, and virtually anyone else who wants to buy the data.

How can you protect the privacy of your medical records? Follow these tips from the Privacy Right Clearinghouse at the Center for Public Interest Law, University of San Diego:

[2]Leah R. Garnett, *"An Open Book,"* Harvard Health Letter 20, no. 11 (September 1995): 1.

- Revise blanket waivers by crossing out sections that authorize all providers to release everything in your medical records. Specify that you are allowing the release of records covering treatment of a specific condition by a particular hospital or doctor.

- Your medical records become part of the public record if they are subpoenaed for a legal proceeding. Ask the court to open only a specific portion of the record or to keep it closed. After the case is decided, you can also ask the judge to seal your medical information.

- If you want your doctor to withhold certain information from your insurance company or employer, say so in writing and pay for the visit yourself. You may even want to consult a different physician and pay the bill.

These additional suggestions were given in the June 1996, Volume 15, Number 3, *People's Medical Society Newsletter* and are reprinted with permission:

- Inform your doctor that you will authorize the release of information about your health on a case-by-case basis only. You may want your records released to your new health insurance carrier but not to a marketing firm that compiles statistics on individuals with specific diseases, for example.

- When you enter the hospital, don't sign any blanket releases that may allow your records to be disseminated far and wide. If the hospital is a teaching hospital, remember that you have the right to refuse to allow a student, intern, or resident to treat you. Likewise, you can object to their reading your medical records.

- When you apply for health or life insurance, supply only the information necessary to obtain the policy. The insurance industry gathers medical information gleaned from policy applications and claims and stores it in a central data bank for future reference. To find out if the industry's Medical Information Bureau has a file on you, contact them at (617) 426-3660.

- Be cautious of supplying personal medical information at health fairs and screenings. Hospital and pharmaceutical marketers often use information gathered at such events to generate a marketing base.

HOSPITAL SCHEDULES (AND WHY THEY ARE THAT WAY)

Traditionally, hospital schedules have been set up for the efficiency of the doctors and the hospital staff. The shifts change at 7:00 A.M., 3:00 P.M., and 11:00 P.M. in most hospitals. That's why you'll often be awakened by breakfast trays being delivered at 6:00 to 6:30 A.M. so the patients will have eaten before the doctors make their rounds at 7:00 to 7:30 A.M. While it is effective for the physicians and staff, the noise and bustle in the early hours often add to the disorientation overtaking those who are seriously ill as well as many elderly patients who are hospitalized and are now jolted out of their regular routine.

One adult child, noting her elderly mother's growing confusion and withdrawal while she was hospitalized, insisted that her mother be permitted to sleep until the physician arrived for his rounds. Then the mother was served what had been her standard breakfast for her sixty-five adult years—coffee and toast—around 10:00 A.M. Yes, it involved more work and attention by the staff, but it resulted in a calmer, more coherent patient, one who then was able to take a more active part in her treatment plan and who moved rapidly on the road to recovery.

VOLUNTEERING FOR A RESEARCH PROJECT

What if you have the opportunity to volunteer for a research project? The operative word here, of course, is "volunteer." Research projects are the backbone of advances in medicine. Without proper testing first with laboratory animals and then with volunteer human subjects, new treatments and medications would never be developed. As with any type of experimentation, however, the outcome cannot be guaranteed.

Research has become big business. Researchers get money for their projects from the government as well as interested parties, such as pharmaceutical companies, nonprofit patient organizations, and the hospitals or universities where they are employed, in order to develop new procedures and medications. There are strict regulations for testing medications—including running double-blind studies where half of the subjects (animal or human) receives the actual drug and the other half receives something that resembles the same drug, but isn't (called a placebo). To prevent the researchers' expectations from skewing the results, double blind studies are also performed where neither the researcher nor the subject knows who received the actual drug and who the placebo.

Subjects for research projects should be carefully selected to fit whatever precise criteria is required of each. It could be subjects all of the same age, same stage of the disease, ethnic background, gender, etc. And, as the above Patients' Bill of Rights lists in number 10, patients must be fully informed in order to give their consent.

While informed consent sounds as though it should be a given, it often isn't. In 1990, three Florida women filed a lawsuit claiming that at least thirty-five research experiments to determine whether steroids would improve their premature babies' lung development were performed on them while pregnant. Part of the experiment included submitting to frequent amniocentesis, a procedure in which amniotic fluid from the uterus is withdrawn by use of a large needle inserted through the mother's abdomen into the uterus. Complications from this procedure include a

1 percent risk of spontaneous abortion, stillbirth or premature delivery, bleeding, infection, or injury to the fetus.

Although the experimental outcome was successful, the women filing the lawsuit said they signed the consent form while still groggy from medications, did not understand what they were signing, and were given consent forms written in English although they spoke Spanish.

According to their lawyer, "They were given a three-page single-spaced document that a sophomore in college might be able to figure out, but even then it doesn't have the information federal law demands to be in there about risks and alternatives."[3]

A federal judge has since ruled that all pregnant women who are or had been part of the study since November 1986 could be included in the suit, possibly bringing the numbers well into the hundreds or even thousands.

INFORMED CONSENT

Informed consent means that you understand and give permission for a procedure (including anesthesia) to be conducted on you, even though there could be complications (including death) resulting from it. Informed consent consists of three steps, all of which must be fulfilled in order for you to have given it.

1. The procedure and its attendant risks must be carefully explained to you while you are mentally alert, not sedated or under the influence of pre-op medications.

2. Anything you do not understand must be re-explained to you in such a way that you comprehend what is being said.

3. You and the person explaining the procedure must sign the consent form in front of a witness.

[3]Cathy Cummins, "Pregnancy Suit's Scope Still to Be Determined," The Tampa Tribune, 29 March 1996, Florida/Metro section.

This can be a very frightening experience because every possible risk must be explained to you, even though it rarely happens. Nevertheless, if serious side effects occur in 1 percent of the cases, you could be that 1 percent, so pay attention.

If you haven't done so before, ask how many of these procedures the individual doing them has performed and what the outcome was. If, as is commonly the case in a teaching hospital, the doctor has observed many such procedures, but yours is the first one he or she has actually done, beware. Obviously, someone has to be the first, but do you want it to be you?

Remember, you have the right to insist that *your* physician or surgeon do the procedure, rather than a resident. You also can refuse to have the procedure observed by medical students and residents, if you so choose.

This principle of informed consent is so important that the American College of Surgeons, the largest organization of surgeons in the world with nearly 52,000 members, suggests asking your proposed surgeon these following questions before granting permission for any surgical procedure:

1. What are the indications that lead you to the opinion that an operation is necessary?

2. What, if any, alternative treatments are available for my condition?

3. What will be the likely result if I don't have the operation?

4. What are the basic procedures involved in the operation?

5. What are the risks?

6. How is the operation expected to improve my health or quality of life?

7. Is hospitalization necessary and, if so, how long can I expect to be hospitalized?

8.   What can I expect during my recovery period?

9.   When can I expect to resume normal activities?

10.   Are there likely to be residual effects from the operation?

Although your surgeon should volunteer much of this information, don't hesitate to ask these or additional questions before signing the consent form. Obviously, no doctor can, or should, guarantee the outcome, because each operation is different, depending on the individual condition and response of each patient. Nonetheless, your surgeon can give you a good idea of what to expect. If, however, he or she just says, "Oh, don't worry about anything," start worrying.

WITH RIGHTS COME RESPONSIBILITIES

Patients and their families are becoming ever more aware of a patient's rights and are acting on this knowledge, thanks in part to the spread of this information through the popular press. Yet seldom do we hear about a patient's obligations that come along with these rights.

Among these inherent responsibilities are listening to what is being said to you by the medical staff, asking questions if you don't understand or if you feel a mistake is being made, and answering questions asked of you honestly and completely. Most physicians and hospital staff want to help their patients; otherwise, they probably would have gone into less stressful professions (and thereby spent more time with their families). Patients who withhold information or who lie (about drinking or drug habits, discomfort or compliance, age or weight) not only undermine the health professional's ability to treat the patient properly, but also, in many cases, subject themselves to unnecessary dangers.

Some medications are administered according to weight. Falsifying your weight may save your ego at the expense of your life. Withholding information about an addiction to alcohol or drugs or hiding the fact that you are a smoker can have deadly implications, especially if you are going under a general anesthetic.

Create a Living Will

It is your responsibility to let your physician know your wishes pertaining to your medical care. You can do so through a living will, which is a legal document through which you express your wishes for medical treatment if you are unconscious, near death, or otherwise unable to communicate your preferences. It specifies your instructions as to whether or not you want your life to be prolonged by artificial means if you are in a terminal state.

Through your living will you should carefully pick and choose exactly what you do and do not want done to you if you become terminally ill. For example, you could say "no" to cardiopulmonary resuscitation (CPR), "no" to a respirator, "yes" to nutrition and hydration (food and water) or "no" to nutrition and "yes" to hydration, and so on. In many states, if you do not specifically declare otherwise, nutrition and hydration will continue to be given to you (by a feeding tube) even if all other life support measures have stopped.

Remember that your decisions are not set in stone. If, while you are lucid or become conscious again, you decide that you would prefer that CPR be tried at least once or you would desire hydration, you can make those changes. What you thought you wanted before, while you were still healthy, may not be your choice now, when you are ill or having surgery and the choice is not so theoretical.

State law varies as to whether or not the living will is legally binding. According to experts at Choice in Dying (1-800-989-WILL), at present no legislation has been written in Michigan or New York, but even in these states, case law supports a living will. Alabama and Alaska are two states that do not currently have legislation in place authorizing the appointment of a health-care agent to make end-of-life decisions. Unfortunately, some physicians will disregard your expressed wishes regardless. Once you have created your living will, discuss your choices with your physician. If he or she feels unable to follow your wishes, seek another doctor who will.

Create a Health-Care Power of Attorney

The health-care power of attorney, like the living will, is a legal document. Also called "health-care proxy," "health-care surrogate," or "attorney-in-fact," it authorizes someone of your choosing to make medical decisions for you if you are unable to. If and when you are able to take control of decisions pertaining to your medical care, you may do so.

This person should be someone who will listen to your feelings and remember your views on quality-of-life issues. He or she will have to make medical choices for you based on *your* values, not his or her own. Sometimes this is much more difficult than it may seem, especially when other friends or relatives add their own personal thoughts to the mix.

Although most people select a spouse or relative to be their health-care proxy, it need not be. You cannot, however, select your physician or the physician's employee or relative, an employee of the hospital or the employee's relative, or someone who is guardian of your property, unless that person is also your legal guardian.

Advanced Directive

"Advanced directive" is the term for both the living will and the health-care power of attorney. These two legal documents keep you in control of your medical care, even when you are unconscious or otherwise unable to communicate your wishes. Depending upon how the legislation was written, in many states, these documents are legally in effect anytime you are unable to express yourself, such as under general anesthesia, and not only in terminal situations.

You don't need an attorney to prepare these documents, both of which can be altered or canceled at any time. State laws vary, but most require the signatures of two adult witnesses, at least one of whom cannot be a spouse, blood relative, heir to your estate, or responsible for paying your medical bills. Often, a notary is required as well.

To learn the requirements of your particular state, contact your local bar association, medical association, or the "Choice in Dying" organization. Organized twenty-five years ago, this latter group can give you the living-will and health-care power-of-attorney forms for your particular state. Send $3.50 to "Choice in Dying," 200 Varick Street, New York, NY 10014 or call them toll-free at 1-800-989-9455.

Understanding a Do Not Resuscitate (DNR) Order

Although this is a book about how to get out of the hospital alive, there may come a time when you aren't going to. We firmly believe that you have the right to make the decision to say, "Enough already" or as one woman's ill and elderly mother phrased it the day before she died, "I gave it a pretty good run for my money, didn't I?"

If you have included those instructions in your living will, you (if you're able at that time) or your assigned spokesperson should check to be sure that DNR (do not resuscitate) has been conspicuously marked on your medical chart. That means you do not want cardiopulmonary resuscitation, to have your heart restarted. A study reported in a November 1995 issue of the *Journal of the American Medical Association* revealed that 49 percent of those wanting no CPR did *not* have that fact written on their chart. Unfortunately, even though you may have recorded that request and told your physician of your preference, some doctors may still disregard your wish and you'll find yourself back in the midst of things even after saying all of your good-byes.

An Ethics Committee and Its Function

The ever-growing technological aspect of medicine has created numerous ethical issues never before faced by health-care professionals or families. There are far more gray areas, with varied possible answers to a single question. To help with this dilemma, the Joint Commission on Accreditation of Healthcare Organizations (JCAHO) has mandated that all organizations seeking accreditation have a "mechanism for the consideration of ethical issues arising in the care of patients" and "provide education to caregivers *and* patients on ethical issues."

Today, many hospitals now have a functioning Ethics Committee, a trained multidisciplinary group of health-care professionals, including numerous physician specialists, nurses, social workers, lay members of the community, clergy, and often an ethics consultant. In most instances, any member of the medical staff, health-care professional, patient, or family member can request a consultation or case review by appropriate members of the Ethics Committee. Ask if your hospital has such a group and how it is convened, if needed.

Although the patient advocate can request a consultation by the ethics committee and will have the opportunity to speak up and explain the patient's side of the issue, he or she usually is not permitted to sit in while the ethics committee assembles to make its decision.

How Hospice Helps

Sometimes, the reason you want to get out of the hospital alive is so that you can go home to die. This home health care for the terminally ill is called hospice care. (There also are hospice facilities in some hospitals, and free-standing hospice centers.) In the past twenty years, more patients are turning their backs on high-tech impersonal death and have been asserting their right to die at home, surrounded by their loved ones.

Using hospice care doesn't mean, however, that you are abandoning your right to medical care. The goal has just shifted from searching for a cure to providing comfort. You still can receive palliative treatment and be free from pain. Often, family members can be trained by hospice nurses to help with your care, including giving injections, suctioning tubing, flushing ports, and helping to make you more comfortable. Home care workers and hospice nurses, therapists, and other staff will be available to stop in each day to check on you. These dedicated individuals are trained, not only to care for your physical needs, but also to provide counseling and bereavement support for you and your entire family.

While there is a national hospice organization with local chapters in many communities, other groups, such as religious organizations, also provide hospice-type terminal care. Your doctor may hesitate to suggest hospice care, because to do so would be admitting that there is little chance for a cure or remission. (Hospice care is usually offered to patients with six months or less to live.)

Some physicians, forgetting that we all are mortal, consider terminal patients a failure on their part, a reminder that they were unable to cure them. Sometimes, these doctors neglect visiting their dying patients, unable to face them. If your doctor doesn't suggest hospice or seems uncomfortable when you bring up the subject, contact the hospital social worker or a member of the clergy. Ask for a referral to a hospice-care program in your area.

Most private and federal health-insurance policies, including Medicare and in many states Medicaid, now provide for hospice care. Check with your insurance provider.

While dying at home can be a traumatic and emotional process, for the patient as well as the family members, it also can be a special and loving experience. Most of the people whose loved ones are able to care for them at home report a sense of comfort and relief and feel closer to their family than at any other time in their lives. They are able to say meaningful good-byes. This is true for the family members as well. Children and teenagers tend to feel less shut out of the process than they would if the person

---

☞   While the decision of where to die is yours whenever possible, there are certain factors you should consider before determining if you want to go home for your last days.

- *Will you feel comfortable having family members caring for your personal physical needs?*

- *Do you have a good emotional relationship with family members? Former resentments and tensions may still be present on both sides, despite your weakened medical condition.*

- *Is your primary caregiver willing and able (physically and emotionally) to provide for your care?*

- *Does your community have visiting nurses, home health-care professionals, a hospice, respite facilities, and other services that can make dying at home easier—for you as well as your family?*

- *Will your family respect your wishes and follow your lead, allowing you to discuss your death if you so desire and refraining from doing so if you don't want to talk about it?*

---

was in the hospital. This makes them more able to accept the reality of death as a natural part of life's circle.

In his book, *Peace, Love & Healing,* surgeon-author Bernie S. Siegel, M.D., writes, " . . . dying can be a healing, ending a full, rich life for someone who is tired and sore and in need of rest. More important, the knowledge of our eventual death is what gives meaning, urgency and beauty to every day of our lives."[4]

We agree.

---

[4]*Bernard S. Siegel,* Peace, Love & Healing *(New York: Harper & Row, 1989), 234.*

CHAPTER 7

Diagnostic Procedures

"A few simple tests." That's what patients are often told they must undergo when they're admitted to the hospital. The truth is, there are really very few "simple" tests. Many of them are invasive. That means that in order to perform the test, the doctor or technician must insert or inject a needle, tubing, dye, or other chemical substance into your body. In addition to possible pain or discomfort, you may suffer from:

- An allergic reaction, which could vary from itching to an inability to breathe or death

- Internal bleeding, which sometimes is difficult to locate or stop

- An inadvertent puncture of a nearby artery, intestine, or other organ

- Infection

Even the so-called "simple" test of amniocentesis, to which thousands of pregnant women are subject, carries with it the risk of miscarriage. According to one study, one out of 200 women suffers a miscarriage after having an amniocentesis. Does that mean that the procedure should be stopped? We think not, because in many cases, the amniocentesis test is done to determine whether or not a women is carrying a baby with a serious genetic abnormality such as Down's syndrome or spina bifida.

However, if the parents would not consider the possibility of terminating the pregnancy if the fetus were seriously affected, perhaps they should reconsider the wisdom of having the procedure. There's no reason to have an invasive procedure of any kind if the results would not alter a treatment decision.

It's impossible to list all the medical procedures that may possibly be prescribed for you while you're in the hospital. Even if we could, because of expanding technology, new procedures would be devised between the time we write this section and the time the book is published.

Regardless of the procedure, however, certain information is vital for you to obtain before agreeing to have any type of test, especially those that are invasive or have any possible harmful side effects. Before signing any consent form for a diagnostic procedure or moving onto the gurney or wheelchair, always ask these questions:

- Who is this test for? (It's not as silly a question as it may seem. The procedure may be intended for your roommate or Mr. Geoffrey Ralph and you're Mr. Ralph Geoffrey.)

- What is the purpose of this procedure?

- Why do you need the information you hope to gain?

- Can the information be obtained any other way?

- What preparation, if any, is required?

- How is the procedure conducted?

- Will it be painful or uncomfortable? (Remember, pain is subjective. What the doctor calls "just a pinch" may be excruciating to you.)

- Who conducts the test?

- How much experience have they had doing this procedure?

- What will I feel during the test?

- What are the possible side effects of the dye, barium, or other chemicals used in the testing procedure?

- How long should these side effects last?

- Will I be subjected to radiation?

- Is there another, less painful (dangerous, expensive) way to get the same information?

- Is this test really necessary?

- What happens if I *don't* have this procedure?

Even the simplest of procedures carries with it attendant risks, most of which are never explained to the patient or the family. In this section we describe numerous procedures, telling how and why they are done along with what can go wrong. Asking questions, such as those listed above, and identifying yourself (or the patient) by asking, "Is this for (give your name)?" is strongly suggested. Errors in giving the right test to the wrong patient are common.

This is not to say that all of the problems that arise in a hospital are due to human error, so don't reach for the phone to call your son-in-law, the lawyer. Just as people are different in appearance, there also are internal variances. A femoral artery, sometimes used to deliver chemotherapy as well as dye in various test procedures, may actually wind its way through the leg uniquely in different individuals. Similarly, a person's heart may lie slightly askew, not conforming to the usual profile. Some individuals are born with one kidney, a fact often unknown until a problem arises. These alterations in what is considered "normal" may create

---

Remember, you *always* have the right to refuse any procedure.

challenges for medical personnel charged with carrying out various procedures.

Although you can't do anything about your anatomy, you need to be aware what precautions you should take before undergoing any medical procedure and become knowledgeable about what medications have been prescribed for you.

Back in the 1960s, when women who had just given birth were permitted to remain in the hospital for at least three to five days, a new mother discovered she was the only woman in the maternity ward nursing her baby. A nurse walked in with little white pills in a paper cup.

"What are they for?" the mother asked.

"They're to dry you up," the nurse responded. "Just take them."

"But I'm nursing my baby," the new mother explained. "This happened every four hours during my entire stay," the woman recalled. "If I hadn't been alert, I would have taken their pills and then wondered why I couldn't breast-feed my baby." She paused. "Maybe that's what they had in mind."

It's impossible to stress too much how important it is to know the names of medications you are given, along with the proper dosage, frequency, and potential side effects. Many patients and their families never know the names of any medications handed to them. Patients, especially those who are elderly and not used to questioning authority, may be especially hesitant to make a fuss and may meekly swallow whatever pill or liquid is handed to them, despite having just taken the same medication or not realizing that they are taking something meant for the person in the next bed. Children need to have an adult family member with them to monitor medications to prevent mistakes as well.

The patient must become a full partner of the health-care team. As the late Norman Cousins wrote in *Anatomy of an Illness,* ". . . the patient is a powerful partner. When of legal age and competent, no decision can be made, treatment begun or changed apart from the patient's consent. Moreover, decisions by the patient must reflect 'informed consent.' Technically, this notion of informed consent implies that the patient receives more than a warning of inherent risks. Information should describe alternative treatments and in a clear enough fashion that lifestyle projections can be made for each possible choice."

Yes, it takes time to carry out this task, a gift few harried nurses enjoy. Physicians, often required by health insurance companies to see the maximum number of patients in a minimal amount of time, may be frustrated by requests for this information. Don't be bullied by a doctor's impatience or feel embarrassed to request and demand this information. It's easier than you may think. Practice saying some of these openers:

"Doctor, before you go, I need to ask you two questions." Then pick up your pad of paper or turn on a tape recorder, if you brought one. (This makes it difficult for most physicians to scurry out the door without pausing to answer just two questions.)

"Mrs. Barkley, this doesn't look like my Procardia. Would you check the PDR to be sure. I know neither of us wants to make a mistake." (The fact that you know what a *Physician's Desk Reference* [PDR] is may give the nurse pause. The statement that you are helping her to correct a possible mistake will urge her to take action.)

"What medication are you putting in my IV line and what is it for? What side effects might I feel?" (Write the answer down on your notepad. Ask the nurse for the correct spelling, if necessary.)

These are assertive questions, not aggressive. It is your right as a patient to ask these and others pertaining to your well-being. Your life may depend on the answers you'll receive. It's your body.

Why do doctors require so many tests? In 1983, George D. Lundberg, M.D., wrote an article for the prestigious *Journal of the American Medical Association* called "Perseveration of Laboratory Test Ordering: A Syndrome Affecting Clinicians," which was based on a study by B.G. Wertman, S.V. Sostrin, and Z. Pavlova.[1] In it, he

---

[1] G.D. Lundberg, M.D. *"Perseveration of Laboratory Test Ordering: A Syndrome Affecting Clinicians,"* Journal of the American Medical Association *249, no. 5 (4 February 1983): 639.*

described the reasons physicians order the number of tests they do. The list is as pertinent today as it was then. As you'll notice, not all of the motives have anything to do with you, the patient. The impetus includes:

Confirmation of clinical opinion	*CYA (Covering Your Ass)*
Diagnosis	*Documentation*
Monitoring	*Personal profit*
Screening	*Hospital profit*
Prognosis	*Attempt to defraud*
Unavailability of prior result	*Research*
Previous abnormal result	*Curiosity*
Question of accuracy of prior result	*Insecurity*
Patient-family pressure	*Frustration at having nothing else to do*
Peer pressure	*Buy time*
Pressure from recent articles	*Hunting or fishing expeditions*
Personal reassurance	*Establish a baseline*
Patient-family reassurance	*Complete a database*
Public relations	*Personal education*
Ease of performance with ready availability	*Report to an attending physician*
Hospital policy	*Habit*
Legal requirement	*Others*
Medicolegal need	

The worst offenders of this policy, of course, are found in the teaching hospitals where medical students, PGY1s (stands for "first year post graduate" or what we used to call "interns"), and residents alike use test results to make their diagnoses, rather than taking time they don't have to listen to what the patient says and carefully improving their own powers of observation.

These extra tests, repeated endlessly, increase the costs of hospitalization, may cause pain, discomfort, or unnecessary exposure to radiation, and encourage errors in conducting and reading the results because the technicians are overworked as a result of the redundancy.

What's more, many test results are false—either giving a false positive or a false negative. A false positive can move you onto the conveyor belt of additional and often invasive procedures; a false negative, of course, can kill you, as those whose Pap tests and other cancer slides were mistaken for negative when they actually were positive could tell you—if they were still alive to do so.

What can you do to prevent unnecessary tests? Speak up, rather than blindly submitting. Ask if the physician would administer the test to a parent or spouse under the same circumstances. Remember, many doctors prescribing these tests for you have never had to experience them. They don't know what it's like, for example, to take a series of enemas to clean your bowel out before having a "simple" sigmoidoscopy. They've never swallowed a "barium cocktail" (despite being mixed with chocolate, it *still* tastes like chalk) in order to have an upper GI X-ray series. Maybe medical school students and residents should be required to undergo a few of these procedures before being permitted to order them on others.

There are risks to most testing procedures. While some may be relatively mild, others can be very serious and potentially fatal. People have suffered massive heart attacks having "routine" stress tests on treadmills. If you are one of those extremely allergic to the dye used in various kidney and neurological tests, the fact that death is a rare side effect will do little to cheer up your grieving family. A "simple" colonoscopy can be uncomfortable; if the doctor doing the procedure perforates your colon, it can be extremely painful and potentially fatal.

Obviously, many of these tests, such as the colonoscopy, can also be lifesaving if a tumor is discovered in time for you to receive treatment before the cancer has spread. We're not saying don't have these tests, only that you should just have the ones you really need and take time beforehand to be certain that the person performing the procedures is experienced and well-trained.

Generally, you are better off having as few tests as possible. Just because we have the technology to run them doesn't mean you need to volunteer to help pay for the new machine, satisfy the doctor's curiosity, or add one more "case study" for a research project unless you understand that you are part of a study, have been fully informed, and have signed a permission statement.

Remember, too, that many physicians today are concerned (rightly so) about being sued by their patients, so they practice what is called "defensive medicine," ordering a variety of unnecessary tests so that, if needed, they can testify in court that they had thought of every possibility in making their diagnosis. According to a recent study by the AMA, defensive medicine costs Americans well over $20 billion annually. While it may be defensive for the doctors, we patients are the ones being tackled—with soaring medical costs, sometimes painful and even harmful tests, and occasionally, needless death.

Common Tests and Procedures

"Just say no" seems to be a good slogan here. Say no to testing procedures unless the doctors can answer all your questions and quiet your fears.

We'll describe the specifics of what you should know about a variety of common testing procedures below, including necessary preparation, how the procedure is performed, what the desired result or outcome is, and what problems can occur.

☞ Be assertive and offer information about your medical condition before you submit to any of these procedures. Never assume the physician or technician already knows your medical history. Something important may have been omitted, such as the fact that you *could* be pregnant, are taking medications (prescription or over-the-counter), had coffee and a doughnut rather than fasting, or have a breast implant. Even if you don't consider this information to be vital, it could be, so mention it. If you are the caregiver to a child or elderly relative, write all the pertinent information down so *you* don't forget.

If you feel that your physician has ordered a number of procedures without apparent cause or sufficient explanation for you, or has performed them and still doesn't know what's wrong, or you think that he or she may be missing something, ask for a second opinion. (Bring copies of all the test results with you.) A colleague may have the answer without subjecting you to a number of additional invasive procedures, which carry with them some potentially dangerous side effects. If your doctor doesn't propose the idea of bringing in a consultant, you do it. Your physician may feel (wrongly) that to suggest he or she needs help is a sign of weakness. It isn't, of course. It's the admission of being wise enough to know that none of us has all the answers.

Angiography

A test in which a solution that shows up on X rays is injected into blood vessels in order to check for abnormalities. A small percentage of people (less than 1 percent) is allergic to the dye. Other possible complications include cardiac arrest (less than 1 percent chance), arrhythmia, and infection from the arterial puncture (less than 1 percent of patients experience this).

Angioplasty

The inflation of a balloon-like device into a narrowed artery for the purpose of dilating the vessel. Complications may include a 1 to 5 percent chance of perforation of the artery, bleeding, or infection.

Arthroscopy

Examination of the inside of a joint, such as the knee, by using a thin optical instrument. Surgery often is performed using the same technique. While there are few complications, there is a less than 1 percent chance of bleeding or bacteria entering the puncture site and causing infection.

Biopsy

Any surgical procedure in which a small sampling of bodily tissue is removed to study under a microscope to determine whether or not it is malignant. In addition to the possibility of bleeding, this procedure makes the body more vulnerable to infection. The amount and location of tissue selected are vital, because there needs to be enough sampling for one or more tests to be run. The swipe also may take unaffected tissue and miss the site of malignant cells. Accurate results also depend upon the skill of the technician reading the slides.

Bronchoscopy

This is one of many types of endoscopies, all of which are used for diagnostic purposes. In this procedure, a thin, flexible tube called a bronchoscope is passed down the anesthetized throat in order to visualize the major air passages of the lungs. Although complications occur in less than 1 percent of the cases, they do exist and may include perforation, bleeding, swelling, and infection.

Carotid Arteriograms

A procedure in which a special dye is injected into the carotid artery in the neck to check for possible blockage. X rays are taken as the dye moves through the blood vessels into the brain. This procedure is used as a diagnostic tool when someone has suffered a stroke or has other abnormalities. Complications include a 1 percent chance of bleeding, a 2 to 3 percent chance of blot clots or triggering a stroke, and a less than 1 percent chance of possible infection.

CAT Scan (Also Known as Computerized Axial Tomography)

This is a painless diagnostic procedure in which multiple X-ray pictures are taken of the head or other parts of the body, and processed by a computer, which illustrates details in slice-like views. Tumors and hemorrhages show up on the film as shadows, which enable the physician to detect the size and location of a lesion. If contrast studies are needed, a dye is injected into a vein. Less than 1 percent of patients are allergic to the dye. You are exposed to some radiation with this procedure.

CBC and Other Blood Tests

CBC stands for "complete blood count." A great deal can be determined by this test, including whether you have an infection (higher than normal white count) and whether you are anemic, which would be determined by too low a red cell count.

Other blood tests include the "smack" (SMA, or sequential multiple analyzer), which shows the balance and percentages of your body's chemicals, and various specialized tests that reveal the possible presence of cancer. Additional blood studies show your blood clotting time.

The most common complications arising from blood work are infection from the wound and the puncturing of a vein or artery. Usually, the complaints are that the technician "poked around" without finding a vein and that too many blood tests are being taken, rather than all studies being done from one sampling.

Although most blood for these tests is drawn from a vein in the crook of your arm, it occasionally is taken from the finger in what is known as a "finger stick," in which a small blade or needle pokes the finger and the blood is squeezed onto a glass slide. If this is done, offer a finger on your nondominant hand. Your dominant hand is usually used for what is euphemistically referred to as "personal hygiene" (i.e., wiping yourself after using the toilet), and the open wound in your finger could become infected.

Cardiac Catheterization

This diagnostic procedure is carried out under a local anesthetic. A flexible tube is fed into a blood vessel in your groin and into your heart in order to check the heart's anatomy. Although you will be given some sedation, you may feel slight pain and, as dye is released to illustrate the size of the opening in your artery, you may experience a flushing sensation. Complications may include puncturing the vessel, infection, bleeding, allergy to the dye, dislodging a clot, and triggering a stroke.

Colonoscopy

This procedure examines the entire length of the inside of the colon (large intestine) in order to check for unexplained blood in the stool, suspected colon cancer, abnormal finding on a lower GI X ray (barium enema), removal of a polyp or small growth (known as a "polypectomy"), or as a follow-up examination for patients with certain intestinal diseases, such as ulcerative colitis. It is done with a six-foot-long flexible tube inserted through the anus.

Complications from this procedure include a perforation of the colon (occurs in 1 out of 500 patients not having a polyp removed). Other complications may include bleeding, abscess formation, lacerations of the rectum, and (rarely) explosion of bowel gas with electrocautery. When polypectomies are performed, the incidence of bleeding is about 2 percent, and perforation occurs in approximately 1 out of 350 cases. Be sure that the gastroenterologist (intestinal specialist) or surgeon performing your colonoscopy is well-trained and well-experienced in performing this procedure.

Cystoscopy

A diagnostic procedure in which a lighted tube is inserted through the urethra in order to visually examine the interior of the bladder. It also may be used to burn out polyps. Complications of less than 1 percent may include bleeding, puncture of the urethra or bladder, and introduction of bacteria leading to infection.

Dilation and Curettage (D&C)

This is one of the most frequently performed surgical procedures, with 1 of every 200 American women having a D&C each year. It is done for a variety of reasons, including abnormal uterine bleeding, bleeding after menopause, removal of remaining placenta after delivery, and abnormal cells on a Pap smear. It includes the dilation of the cervix and the scraping of the lining of the womb.

A D&C is performed under a general or local anesthetic, with all the attending risks that anesthesia entails. Complications are less than 1 percent and include possible perforation of the uterus, bleeding, the introduction of bacteria into the body, and a high incidence of false-negative (above 15 percent) diagnoses of cancer.

Gastrointestinal Series: Upper and Lower

The procedure known as "upper GI" is a diagnostic test to check for cancer, ulcers, polyps, and abnormalities of the upper intestinal tract. A barium drink is swallowed and its progress noted as it passes through the esophagus, stomach, and duodenum by using fluoroscope and X ray. Complications include a great deal of radiation from the fluoroscope, which is ongoing, unlike the instant exposure from an X ray. There also is a 2 to 3 percent possibility of barium impaction, which blocks the bowel if the individual doesn't drink adequate water to flush it out.

The study of the large intestine is called "lower GI series." In this procedure, the barium is inserted through the rectum by an enema.

Intravenous Line

The intravenous line, also known as IV, is a thin plastic tube inserted with a needle into a vein—usually on the back of your hand or in the fold of your arm opposite your elbow. The other end of the tube attaches to a bottle or plastic bag that hangs from a metal pole over or beside your bed. The bottle or bag contains chemicals, medications, saline, or nutrients, which slowly drip into your vein.

The IV needle should be placed in your nondominant hand or arm. Sometimes your hand or arm is attached to a splint to prevent your bending your arm or wrist. Nevertheless, having it in your nondominant hand or arm may keep you from moving that limb as much as if it were in your dominant arm.

Always ask what is in the bag to be sure it is the right contents for the right patient. The bag should be marked with your name, the contents, and the date of expiration. Write the name of the contents and the time you are given it in a notebook. Never allow someone to replace your IV bag without your knowing what you are being given.

Watch for pain, tenderness, swelling, or discoloration at the puncture site of the IV. The needle can slip out of the vein, causing infiltration, which means that the solution that is supposed to be going into your veins is dripping into your subcutaneous tissues instead. This is especially common with older patients whose veins are very fragile and may tear. If the needle has perforated the vein, bleeding will take place as well.

Unfortunately, intravenous lines also may allow bacteria to enter the vein at the puncture site. Tell the nurse at any sign of chills, fever, or just a sense of not feeling quite right. Older patients and those with weakened immune systems are especially vulnerable to this type of nosocomial infection.

For those requiring an IV for some length of time for medication, feeding, or receiving chemotherapy, the IV may be attached to a port, an opening that usually sits in the subclavian vein, up by the collarbone. The port is generally put in by a surgeon, under either general anesthesia or local anesthesia. Although the port is routinely flushed out to keep it open, problems can include infection, secondary hemorrhage, and the clogging of the port. Always ask the nurse to identify any substance he or she injects into your port.

Lumbar Puncture

Also known as a spinal tap, this procedure is used to diagnose injuries and diseases of the nervous system such as meningitis, infections, and tumors. Under a local anesthetic, a needle is inserted between the vertebrae at the base of the spine. You'll feel a brief burning sensation from the anesthetic and pressure when the spinal needle goes in. Tell the doctor immediately if you feel pain, numbness, or a tingling in your legs as that may mean the needle is pressing on a nerve and the physician must relocate the needle.

A small amount of cerebrospinal fluid is removed for study. Complications may include bleeding, fever, sensitivity to light, headache, paralysis, possible infection, and sudden death.

Similar taps are also done to remove fluid from the sac around the lungs (known as a "pleural tap") and from the abdomen (known as "paracentesis").

MRI (Magnetic Resonance Imaging)

This diagnostic scan is conducted to detect abnormalities in the bones, joints, or muscles; possible tumors; disorders of the brain, cardiovascular system, skeletal system, or nervous system; and problems in various major organs. It scans by using a strong magnetic field in combination with radiofrequency waves, rather than radiation.

You'll lie on a narrow metal table in the radiology department. The table moves slowly, carrying you into a cave-like structure, which is the MRI machine. Although there is no sensation during the procedure, you must remain perfectly still for almost an hour or more. Your head, arms, and body may be lightly secured with straps to help you remain motionless. There are loud thumping noises as the magnetic fields are activated, which frighten some people. Others feel anxious and may suffer from claustrophobia from the small enclosure.

Ask the technician for a pillow, if you need one, before the scan begins. You also can request earplugs or earphones with music to drown out the clanking of the machine. If you think you'll have trouble staying motionless or suffer from claustrophobia, ask for a light tranquilizer.

Be sure the doctor knows if you may be pregnant or if you have a pacemaker, aneurysm clip, metal pin, or artifical joint such as a knee or hip replacement. These and other conditions may rule out your having an MRI or require some adjustment on the equipment. Newer MRI equipment is "open," which obviates the claustrophobic side effects.

As radio waves are used with MRI, there is no radiation. If your particular test included the use of a contrast dye to make specific areas stand out, drink plenty of water for the next few days to flush out your system.

Myelogram

The injection of a dye into the spinal canal in order to study the spinal cord and neurological system. You will be exposed to X ray during this diagnostic procedure, so tell the technician if you even think you may be pregnant. Fewer than one percent of patients undergoing this procedure suffer from bleeding, allergy to the dye, or infection.

Paracentesis

The removal of fluid from the abdomen through a needle for both diagnostic and therapeutic reasons. Complications of less than one percent may include hemorrhage, shock, infection, or perforation.

Proctoscopy

This procedure examines the rectum and lower intestine (descending colon) through the use of a lighted scope with an eyepiece at the other end. It is inserted through the anus. It is performed in order to evaluate disorders of the lower colon including rectal bleeding, and in those over forty and in high-risk categories, to screen for colon cancer. Complications are rare, but include bleeding, perforation, and introduction of bacteria.

Protosigmoidoscopy

This diagnostic entails examining the rectum and sigmoid colon with a flexible lighted scope that penetrates further into the colon. Complications are less than 1 percent, but can include perforating the bowel, bleeding, and infection.

Stress Test Without Thallium

This is also called a "Master's Test." It is the serial production of EKGs during and after a known amount of exercise, usually on a treadmill or stationary bike. Readings are taken through electrodes pasted or suctioned to your chest area.

Although the stress test is often given routinely in a physical examination, many physicians believe they should not be ordered without cause. Inaccurate readings can give false positives, suggesting that there is a heart problem when there really isn't one. This can move the patient into other, more invasive testing, which often is unnecessary and which may cause additional complications. Side effects from the stress test alone could include cardiac arrhythmia, pain, shortness of breath, dizziness, nausea, or sudden death.

Stress Test with Thallium

This type of stress test is the same as the previous one described, with the exception that a radioactive isotope called thallium is injected into a vein. After a period of exercise, usually on a treadmill or stationary bike, a radioactive scan is taken to determine blood flow to the heart. Complications of less than 1 percent may include cardiac arrhythmia, pain, shortness of breath, dizziness, nausea, or sudden death.

For more information about these and over 300 diagnostic procedures, read *Everything You Need to Know About Medical Treatments,* written by over fifty leading doctors and medical experts.

CHAPTER 8

Surgery, Surgeons, and Anesthesiologists

lthough numerous procedures done within the hospital setting can have dangerous outcomes, perhaps none is as feared as surgery, sometimes, unfortunately, for good reason. In recent years, the print and electronic media have featured horrendous stories of surgeons at prestigious medical centers mixing up patients' X rays and thereby cutting into the healthy right side of a fifty-nine-year-old woman's brain rather than the left side where the lesion was located; amputating the wrong leg on a fifty-two-year-old diabetic man; removing a fifty-nine-year-old man's healthy lung rather than the diseased one; and inadvertently cutting a uterus of a thirty-three-year-old woman who subsequently bled to death. An eight-year-old boy died during a "routine" ear operation when his anesthesiologist allegedly fell asleep.

According to the People's Medical Society, a nonprofit consumer health organization in Allentown, Pennsylvania, of the 600,000 Americans in the hospital on any given day, 10 to 15 percent will suffer from surgical errors. Why does this happen? More importantly, what can patients and their families do to prevent these mistakes from happening?

According to Thomas Putnam, a retired pediatric surgeon, "Sometimes egos get in the way of good judgment." But it's far more complicated than that. Surgical errors happen for a myriad of reasons—mix-up of X rays and patient charts, surgeons' haste to "beat their time" doing a procedure, poorly trained surgeons, and unnecessary surgeries, especially hysterectomies (nearly half are unnecessary), coronary bypass operations (one out of every three may be unnecessary), and Cesarean sections. In addition, the area of the country in which you live plays an important part in the type of surgery you will undergo. A ten-year study at Dartmouth Medical School revealed that when there is more than one treatment option, doctors make their decision based on local practice. Researchers found, for example, that mastectomies were performed thirty-three times more often than breast-sparing lumpectomies in certain sections of the United States.

How do you know if you really need surgery? How can you find the "right" surgeon? How can you minimize the chances of surgical error while you are anesthetized? How can you speed up your recovery? These are important questions; knowing the correct answers could save your life.

HOW TO KNOW IF SURGERY IS REALLY NECESSARY

Never assume that you need surgery just because the doctor says so. There may be other, more conservative options—and you may not need any type of procedure at all.

A mother took her seven-year-old son to see an orthopaedic surgeon. The boy had webbed toes. The great toe was attached to the next one by a thick cartilage and the second and third toes exited the foot with two bones that merged into one at the tip. The physician suggested surgery to separate the toes.

"Why?" asked the mother.

"Because they're deformed," the physician replied, surprised by her question.

Fortunately, she did ask. With her pediatrician's help, she arranged for a second opinion with a leading pediatric orthopaedist at a major children's hospital. The surgeon observed the little boy as he walked up and down the hall.

"Why would you want to separate his toes?" the doctor asked the parents. "He walks fine."

"Well, the doctor at home . . . " the mother began.

"Is your son self-conscious about having webbed toes?" the doctor interrupted.

"No, not at all," the parents replied in unison.

"Then take him home and forget any operation. There's no reason for it."

That little boy is now thirty-two years old and has had no problems—physically or emotionally—with his webbed toes.

Another example of a proposed unnecessary operation involved a thirty-four-year-old woman who returned to see her obstetrician shortly after giving birth to her fifth child.

"Do you plan any more children?" the doctor asked.

She shook her head. "No, I think we've had our basketball team. We'll have to play without reserves."

"Then maybe you should think about having a hysterectomy."

She looked at her doctor in surprise. "Why? I haven't had any trouble. Why would I have surgery?'

The doctor smiled gently. "It's the best way to keep from getting pregnant that I know of. Besides, then you wouldn't have to worry about ovarian or uterine cancer. Take out the crib, leave the playpen."

Speechless, she shook her head, gathered up her belongings, and walked out.

Neither of these anecdotes involved evil doctors. Actually, both were well respected in their communities and were known for doing good work. Were they overanxious to operate without sufficient cause? A little greedy? Yes, we think so.

Unfortunately, these were not isolated cases. Hysterectomies, which were frequently performed in the nineteenth century supposedly to prevent women from suffering from depression and/or hysteria, are still among the most common types of unnecessary surgery. Nearly half of all hysterectomies performed in the United States are medically unnecessary. According to the People's Medical Society, in 1970 one in twenty babies was delivered by Cesarean section rather than normal vaginal childbirth. Today, one in four babies is delivered by Cesarean section. (Interestingly, both surgeries are performed on women.)

This is not to say that there never is cause for either of these operations. Of course there is. But to advise a hysterectomy as an easy means of contraception or because a woman is past the child-bearing years and "doesn't need a uterus anymore" or doing a Cesarean section for convenience sake and ease of delivery (and to prevent being sued if problems arise connected with the birth), are actions potentially fraught with danger. As a career employee of an ob/gyn office confided, "The doctors always say a Cesarean section is the best way to deliver a baby and minimize the danger to the baby; but it isn't the best way for the mother."

There is no such thing as "minor" surgery. Any surgery—even laparoscopic, which despite seeming simpler to the lay person, actually requires special training and skill—can perforate nearby tissue, trigger bleeding, expose the wound to harmful bacteria, provoke breathing distress, dislodge a blood clot, and cause pain, which thereby exposes you to additional medication, some of which may have adverse effects.

The possibility of surgery will be mentioned to you by either your internist, who suggests you see a surgeon, or by a specialist, who also performs surgery, such as a gynecologist, urologist, or orthopedist. Not infrequently, a potential surgical problem will be discovered in the course of a routine examination, such as a physician discovering a breast lump in an elderly female patient who was being checked to see if she were able to undergo cataract surgery. The first step is to determine whether or not you really require surgery at this particular time in your life. Ask the doctor these questions:

- Why do you think I need surgery?

- Will you explain exactly what type of surgery you're suggesting?

- Are there other, less invasive options I could consider?

- What will happen if I postpone the surgery for a while?

- What will happen if I don't have the surgery at all?

- What benefits will I gain from having this operation?

- What side effects or complications might I expect from this surgery?

- How long will I have to stay in the hospital?

- What could I expect during the recovery period? How long before I could drive, go back to work (be sure the physician understands how strenuous your job is and what it entails), and otherwise fully recover?

- If I were your parent or spouse, would you recommend my having this operation?

If the reasons for surgery seem to be valid to you, seek out a surgeon, if the physician suggesting it doesn't operate. (Even if the doctor does, be sure you're comfortable with him or her as a surgeon, too.) Don't necessarily accept the recommendation given to you by the referring physician. That person may be a good friend, but a mediocre surgeon. You also have to have a comfort level with the person who operates on you. Seeing a surgeon to discuss the possibility of an operation does not mean you have to accept that particular specialist.

How to Find the "Right" Surgeon

Most of us read *Consumer Reports* and similar magazines when we're thinking of buying a new car. We ask friends their opinions, talk to service people at gas stations and garages, check the Internet, and otherwise gather as much information as we can. Why? Because a car's a major purchase, we get emotional about it, and we hope to have it a long time. Why are we often less prudent when it comes to surrendering our body (and, possibly, our life) to someone dressed in blue or green pajamas who wields a very sharp knife?

To paraphrase the Welsh poet Dylan Thomas, "Do not go gently into that surgical suite, but forage, forage (by asking questions) until you know that it's right!"

What makes the "right" surgeon right? It differs for each person. It may not be the man you play golf with—even though he's a great guy. And it may not be the woman you've served with on a number of community committees, despite the fact that she's brilliant, charming, and well-organized.

Begin your research by asking friends, neighbors, and co-workers, especially any who are in the medical field, what experiences they have had with particular surgeons. Call your nearest medical school and hospital to see what surgeons they suggest, although many times the doctors are on a rotating list and you just get the next three names.

Conduct research in the public library, a hospital's medical library, or the medical library of a nearby medical school or medical center. See what papers have been written on the procedure you're about to have and what surgeons' names keep coming up as the "experts" in that particular field. You'll quickly recognize what different procedures are being done for your condition so you'll be better prepared to ask the surgeon why he or she prefers one over another.

If you have a computer and a modem, you can go online to check the World Wide Web. Use the bulletin boards and chat lines on America Online, Prodigy, and CompuServe, too. They're a good way to ask others about their experiences. Remember, however, that no two patients are exactly alike; one may sail through a surgery with no difficulties and the next, even with the same surgeon and identical procedure, experience every complication in the book.

Check the surgeon's credentials with the local medical society. Call the physician's office to see if he or she is board certified. In 1996, for the first time anywhere in the United States, Massachusetts residents were able to receive detailed physician information through a toll-free line. These profiles listed education, awards, hospital associations, as well as whether the doctor had made malpractice settlement payments. At this writing, California offers limited information about doctors to those who call. Florida, Wisconsin, and New York are presently considering opening physician files to their citizens.

Once you've narrowed your list, it's time for a face-to-face meeting with the surgeon. While the final decision of whether to have surgery and who should perform it must be left to the patient, unless he or she is too young, old, ill, or otherwise unable to make that determination, it always is best to have someone with you when you see the surgeon. It is an emotional time, and even if you take wonderful notes and think you're being totally objective, it's difficult to be detached when you are the prospective patient. Many people tape-record the meeting so they can replay it later when they're home and under less stress.

Here are just a few questions you should ask a potential surgeon:

- How many of this type of procedure have you actually done?

  Watching or assisting is not the same as actually doing a procedure, even though it's standard practice in teaching hospitals to train future surgeons. However vital for training, let them practice on your neighbor who hasn't read this book; you want the teacher as your surgeon, not the student. The more often a surgeon has performed a particular operation, the more familiar it (and possible complications) become.

Would you rather fly with an experienced pilot or someone who just soloed?

- What were the outcomes of the procedures you performed, in terms of both mortality and complication rates?

While often used to reassure patients, statistics really don't mean a great deal. Remember that even if there is only a 1 percent fatality rate for a particular procedure, *someone* is part of that 1 percent. If complications are frequent, you need to know. You may still choose to have the surgery, but you should be aware of your survival chances before making that important decision.

- What hospitals do you use?

Often the choice of a particular hospital can affect the outcome of your recovery, due to infection control, patient-staff ratio, and other factors. Be sure the hospital is equipped to handle complications if they should arise, with adequate available technology and experienced staff.

- Tell me what you propose to do, especially why you may want to use a particular technique over another (such as laparoscopic rather than open approach, lumpectomy rather than simple mastectomy, or excising a cyst in the brain rather than having it shunted).

Many surgeons now have videotapes and brochures you can look at that may answer many of these questions or provoke a few more. Often, the surgeon can draw a rough sketch to help explain what he or she plans to do. Don't feel stupid if you still don't understand and don't quit asking questions until you do.

Remember, too, that like all of medicine, surgical techniques evolve. New procedures may be used at major medical centers that have not as yet filtered down through the journals and seminars to all surgeons. Some surgeons may still be using outdated procedures, such as the Halstead radical mastectomy, rather than less invasive simple mastectomy or lumpectomy, where only the tumor and a little surrounding tissue are removed.

Ask what new procedures are currently being done for your particular problem and where they are being performed. At this writing, for example, minimally invasive direct coronary bypass surgery (or "keyhole" surgery) is replacing traditional bypass surgery for selected patients at many hospitals across the country. If a surgeon is up-to-date in reading the extensive literature in the field, he or she will be able to answer your question.

- What should I expect after the anesthesia wears off?

  Knowing this information can reduce fears and anxiety in the recovery room. It also lets you know what is *not* normal so you can immediately report those sensations to the nurse.

- What potential problems could arise?

  Beware of any doctor who says, "Oh, let me handle things. Don't you worry your pretty little head about that." While it doesn't do you any good to worry, you *should* be informed about potential problems so you can alert the nursing staff if any of the difficulties should arise.

  This is especially important if you have other medical conditions that may affect your recovery or increase the possibility of complications. If you have a chronic disorder, such as heart trouble, diabetes, asthma, or cancer, just to mention a few, and are under the care of a specialist, let that physician know before you schedule surgery. He or she may want to consult with the surgeon before or after your operation.

- How long a recovery period should I expect?

  Ask what will be involved during your recovery. If you're having a knee replacement, for example, will you be bed-ridden? Able to use crutches or a walker to go to the bathroom? What about therapy? Can someone come to your home or will you have to go to the therapist? When will you be able to walk? Drive? Exercise? Return to work?

- What will the surgery cost?

  Medical insurance often requires you to be pre-approved before having the surgery. Ask if the surgeon accepts whatever the insurance pays or if you'll be required to pay the remainder. If that presents an extreme hardship, discuss that with the surgeon to see what solution can be worked out. Be sure there are no extra hidden costs.

  Each of the nearly 52,000 members of The American College of Surgeons, the largest organization of surgeons in the world, has taken a Fellowship pledge that says, in part, "I promise to make my fees commensurate with the services rendered and with the patient's rights. . . ." They expect you to ask about fees; do so. Remember that, in addition to the surgeon's fee, you will be billed by the hospital, the anesthesiologist, and any other specialists involved in your care.

- What is your philosophy about pain control?

  Surgeons, like other physicians, vary in their thoughts about controlling pain. At one end of the spectrum are those who feel a little pain is a good thing (on their patients, not themselves). At the other end, however, and often equally harmful, are those who want their patients to experience no sensation of pain at all, and in doing so, may overmedicate a susceptible patient.

  Some physicians now use patient-controlled analgesia (PCA) even on children and find that not only is pain controlled more successfully, but their patients actually used less pain medication than when it is given by the clock. People tend to heal faster when they are relatively pain free.

After your interview with each surgeon, jot down your impressions, reactions, and instincts about him or her as a person. While you obviously want a surgeon who is technically proficient and specialty board–certified, you also need to feel comfortable with this person as an individual. Your life will literally be in his or her hands. You need to sense a rapport, feel that you can communicate effectively, and have a sense of trust. These are intangible requirements, with no objective way to measure them. But they are, nevertheless, very important.

An eighty-year-old woman went to a surgeon for a consultation about her breast cancer. He agreed with her oncologist that she should have a simple mastectomy, which entailed removing the breast but none of the surrounding muscle or lymph nodes. She admitted later to her daughters that she didn't like his abrupt manner, but said nothing and went ahead with the recommended surgery.

After the surgery she returned for a routine check-up. The scar on her chest was uneven and looked as though the remaining skin had been bunched up, wrapped around with string, and tied in knots. The flesh was red and inflamed. "Not too pretty," she remarked sadly.

"What difference does it make?" the surgeon snapped. "You're an old lady." The woman was stunned and fell silent. Her wound remained infected and oozed pus for months, although the surgeon denied there ever was any trace of infection.

Would this patient have fared better with a more compassionate surgeon? Would a healthier emotional state have strengthened her immune system so she might have healed more quickly? We definitely think so. In his many writings, surgeon-author Bernie Siegel describes case after case where empathetic physicians have prolonged the lives of patients that other doctors have termed "hopeless," and, sadly, where other patients have given up and died because the doctor said they would.

Always Get a Second Opinion Before Agreeing to Surgery

Most health insurance programs now (wisely) pay for second opinions concerning surgical procedures because they discovered that operations are not always needed. Some health plans actually *require* a second opinion for all nonemergency surgeries. At this writing, Medicare pays for a second opinion at the same rate it pays for other services. Medicaid programs in most states also pay for a second opinion.

There's no reason ever to feel embarrassed or uncomfortable about telling a surgeon you want to get another opinion. No good doctor is threatened by this type of a request. If the response is "I'm the best and if you want another opinion, you don't want me," which a well-known ear surgeon said to a potential patient, you should answer, "you're right" and leave. Any physician with this kind of arrogance and lack of acceptance for his or her patient's concerns can have too big an ego to ever admit potential trouble if or when it arises in the OR.

We've interviewed a number of top surgeons, the ones who routinely make all the "Best Doctors" lists. These men and women all welcome second opinions because they know that the process eases a potential patient's mind. These physicians understand the dynamics of the mind/body relationship, and know that confidence in both the physician and in the procedure being done plays an important part in speeding the healing process.

Don't ask one of the doctor's partners for a second opinion; chances are they think somewhat alike if they're partners. They also have the bottom line of their practice in common. Instead, check with friends, operating room nurses, other physicians you know and respect, and the hospitals on your medical plan or your local medical association. The latter two groups, however, may only be able to give you a list of physicians who do the particular procedure.

ANESTHESIOLOGISTS

"The gas man's the king," a neurosurgeon confided to us. "He, not me, rules the OR." The tribute, of course, is well-deserved. Anesthesiologists are medical doctors with four years of postmedical school training (one year of internship and three years in an anesthesiology residency program). Many further specialize in a subspecialty, such as neurosurgical anesthesiology, by completing one to two more years in a subspecialty training program.

In many hospitals, nurse anesthetists are part of the anesthesiology team. Nurse anesthetists are registered nurses with two years of specialized training. Although nurse anesthetists cannot prescribe drugs, they administer 65 percent of the 26 million doses of anesthetics delivered annually. In most states, the nurse anesthetist must be supervised by a medical doctor, although it need not be an anesthesiologist.

You can select a particular anesthesiologist, if you've used one previously or have a trusted friend's recommendation. Tell your surgeon early, however, so arrangements can be made. Otherwise, your surgeon will assign one for you.

The anesthesiologist will probably meet with you a day before surgery when you come in for preoperative blood and laboratory tests. If it isn't mentioned that you will meet the anesthesiologist at that time, however, ask for an appointment. You'll probably be less anxious then than right before surgery. In some cases, if you're already in the hospital, you may first see your anesthesiologist the night before surgery. Either way, write down any questions or concerns you may have so you don't forget them.

Keep no secrets from the anesthesiologist. When you have a general anesthesia, you will be totally unconscious and may not be able to breathe on your own. This is the person who will keep you free of pain, control your breathing, keep track of the amount of oxygen in your blood, monitor your blood pressure, measure blood gases, observe your brain and kidney functions, and inject a muscle relaxant to paralyze your muscles. He or she balances a delicate tightrope, keeping you relaxed and pain free without letting your blood pressure drop too low or your breathing stop. After the surgery is completed, the anesthesiologist may administer other drugs to reverse the effects of the previous ones, restore your breathing, and normalize your body's functioning.

In an article "Your Life in My Hands" published by *American Health,* Dr. Andrew G. Kadar, an anesthesiologist on the clinical faculty of the UCLA School of Medicine, writes, "An anesthesiologist's head moves like a submarine periscope, surveying the surgical domain. Is the IV infusing at the proper rate? How is the operation progressing? How much blood loss is there at the wound site, on the sponges and in the suction bottles? What's happening to the patient's heart rate, blood pressure and oxygen saturation? Is ventilation adequate? Do I need to make adjustments in the levels of anesthetic gases? Is the muscle relaxation satisfactory?"[1]

Never lie to your anesthesiologist. Your life literally will be in this person's hands. The anesthesiologist needs to know the truth

---

[1] *Dr. Andrew G. Kada, "Your Life in My Hands,"* American Health *(July/August 1995): 61.*

about your weight and age in order to calculate the correct dosages of the medications you will be given; any drugs you've taken regardless if they're illegal (yes, even report "pot"), prescription or non-prescription (over-the-counter drugs); your alcoholic or smoking habits as they can affect the way an anesthetic drug works on your body; any preexisting medical conditions including (but not limited to) asthma, diabetes, hepatitis, coronary conditions, high or low blood pressure, allergies to drugs, and your previous experiences with anesthesias as well as the previous reactions of blood relatives.

"The average person tends to underestimate his or her alcoholic intake and the number of cigarettes smoked," warns Tampa anesthesiologist Richard Hodes. "Smokers can have post-operative respiratory problems, such as inflammation of the trachea, postop pneumonitis, and partial collapse of the lungs.

"Be forthright about your drinking habits too. Don't say you have one cocktail a night if you actually drink three or four. If you're an alcoholic, say so. Alcoholics have liver damage. As certain anesthesia drugs are not totally metabolized, the by-products can further damage a liver. Alcoholics have a higher tolerance for anesthesia too. That means they need more to get the proper effects; they're also harder to stabilize."

It's important to describe any adverse reactions that you or blood relatives have had under anesthesia as well. Some people have a genetic deficiency of certain enzymes that results in prolonged reactions to specific drugs. These individuals may be difficult to rouse after a general anesthetic. Genetic differences may alter the way a drug is absorbed, metabolized, transported, or excreted. There also may be a family history of malignant hyperthermia, in which, under a general anesthesia, an individual's temperature can suddenly spike to 105°F to 106°F. The patient develops severe muscle rigidity, jaw clenching, and shaking or chilling. Certain drugs can make this condition occur more frequently, especially with children. This situation can be treated during or after surgery, but the anesthesiologist needs to know of its possible existence beforehand.

"Mention something as seemingly minor as a cold or runny nose too, as these conditions could make your airways stuffy," says Murray Canter, M.D., an anesthesiologist at New York University Medical Center. "Ideally, the anesthesiologist should take time to ask you all these questions. But if he or she doesn't, speak up. It's your life."

If you have previously experienced problems with a general anesthesia, there are other methods of anesthesia that might be a possibility for your specific surgery, such as local, regional, and hypnosis. A local anesthesia numbs a small part of your body for a

---

☞ It is your responsibility (or that of your caregiver) to tell the surgeon and the anesthesiologist of any existing medical conditions (such as diabetes, asthma, high or low blood pressure, allergies, and even snoring) that might affect you during or after the surgery. Never assume your surgeon or the anesthesiologist knows of your preexisting medical condition or its severity or has read your chart. A Florida anesthesiologist gave a woman who was in labor an epidural anesthesia despite knowing that she had a heart condition called aortic stenosis that restricted her blood flow. She had a seizure, went into respiratory arrest and cardiac arrest, and died shortly after her baby was delivered by Cesarean section. The anesthesiologist claimed he hadn't realized the severity of her heart condition when he gave the anesthesia and that he had been assured by other physicians that she could tolerate an epidural anesthesia.

Other women have experienced severe falling blood pressure and vomiting with so-called "routine" epidural anesthesias. The rule to remember is that no anesthesia is "routine." Always ask questions and fully inform the anesthesiologist. If you're afraid you won't remember everything, write it down.

Always tell your anesthesiologist if you've been on any type of cortisone—for asthma, colitis, dermatologic conditions, and allergies, for example—for six weeks or longer. If you have been taking cortisone for that length of time, then suddenly stop and have anesthesia, the anesthesiologist may have trouble maintaining your blood pressure. You could start bleeding, have a heart attack, and die of circulatory collapse.

definite period. You probably have experienced this type of anesthesia if you have had a tooth filled or a small wound stitched.

A regional anesthesia—such as a spinal block or an epidural, the latter of which is frequently used today for childbirth—numbs a larger area of your body by blocking the pain receptors from that area to the brain center that registers pain. The medication is injected into the epidural space surrounding the spinal cord. Other areas can be numbed with a regional block. Many surgeons operating to relieve the pain of carpal tunnel syndrome, for example, use a regional anesthesia to numb the hand and wrist area, rather than submitting the patient to the risks of a general anesthesia.

Heed the anesthesiologist's instructions if you've been warned not to eat or drink anything after midnight before surgery. This is not an arbitrary suggestion. You can regurgitate gastric secretions or the contents of your stomach into your lungs under general anesthesia. That can cause aspiration pneumonitis and can burn the lining of your lungs. People die from that. If you take daily medication, ask the anesthesiologist for instructions. Then follow them.

Some anesthesiologists use hypnosis to help patients focus away from the sensation of pain so they require little or no other anesthesia. According to anesthesiologist Richard Hodes, "Hypnosis is often very successful when used in childbirth; it is more difficult to achieve for surgery."

There are risks and side effects with anesthesias, especially if you have additional medical problems. Discuss the pros and cons of each type of anesthesia with the anesthesiologist.

The role of the anesthesiologist doesn't end after surgery is completed. He or she will continue to check on you in the Post Anesthesia Care Unit (PACU), also known as the "recovery room." You will be carefully monitored to be certain you are breathing satisfactorily and that your blood pressure and other vital signs are normal. Only then will the anesthesiologist give permission for you to be taken to your room or special care unit.

When Your Child Needs Anesthesia

Children are not "little adults." Children and adults not only metabolize drugs differently, but they also have airway differences. An anesthesiologist dealing with pediatric patients must understand the effect of anesthesia on tiny lungs and be experienced in administering the proper dosage for a child. That's why you should request a pediatric anesthesiologist if your youngster requires surgery.

A pediatric anesthesiologist also may be used to provide safe mild sedation for your child during diagnostic procedures to help reduce anxiety and to minimize movement, which could affect the accuracy of various tests. He or she also is often involved in providing pain relief for youngsters following surgery or other painful procedures.

In order to help the pediatric anesthesiologist provide the best medication and care for your child, always answer all questions truthfully and to the best of your knowledge. Be sure to include information concerning other medications being taken, any blood relatives who may have had problems with anesthesia, any allergies or other medical conditions your child has (including but not limited to asthma, diabetes, and rheumatic fever), and your child's previous experiences with anesthetics, if any.

Follow the anesthesiologist's instructions to the letter, especially if you're told to give no food and liquids prior to surgery. Even if your child cries and begs for a little something to drink, don't give in if you've been instructed otherwise. Your youngster's life could depend on it. Although many physicians today feel that clear fluids given up to two hours before surgery are safe, never take that course of action without the anesthesiologist's permission.

The Anesthesiologist and Pain Control

The anesthesiologist often is called in to help patients with pain management. There are many treatments for pain control today, not all of which are drugs. For this reason, the anesthesiologist usually heads a team of medical professionals including other physicians, nurses, and therapists.

Pain is not something you need to tolerate after surgery. In fact, it's important to control your pain because it:

- Makes you more comfortable.

- Helps you heal faster because with less pain you are more apt to work at your therapy and do your deep breathing exercises which prevent pneumonia.

- Allows you to get your strength back sooner.

- Makes you less susceptible to pneumonia and blood clots.

Many people hesitate to ask for pain medication because they don't want to be a bother and are afraid of getting "hooked." Studies show addiction is very rare, unless you already have a problem with drug abuse. You should always tell the nurse if you're having pain, because it could be a sign of infection or some other problem related to your surgery. Don't wait until you can't bear the pain anymore to ask for something. Ask for help as soon as the pain starts. If you know the pain will get worse as you start breathing exercises, physical therapy, or walking, take the pain medication first. Once pain takes hold, it's harder to ease it.

Discuss with the anesthesiologist the use of patient-controlled analgesia (PCA). With this method, you control when you get pain medication and don't have to wait for a nurse to answer your call bell. When you begin to feel pain, you press a button to inject the medicine through the intravenous (IV) line into your vein. Studies show that most patients using PCA use *less* pain medications, not more.

Pain treatment may be in the form of medication, given as a pill, injection, suppository, or through a small catheter (tube) in your vein or an area in your back. It also can be a nondrug treatment, such as massage, whirlpool, and ultrasound; hot or cold packs; biofeedback and other relaxation techniques; self-hypnosis, visualization, music, or other distraction methods; and nerve stimulation (TENS, for transcutaneous electrical nerve stimulation).[2]

The latter, according to the American Society of Anesthesiologists, " . . . is the most common form of electrical stimulation. It is not painful and does not require needles. TENS consists of a small, battery-operated device that can stimulate nerve fibers through the skin to diminish pain. Also, electrical stimulation of acupuncture points is sometimes performed."[3]

Two booklets you can order on pain control are:

- "Anesthesia & You . . . The Management of Pain," from the American Society of Anesthesiologists, 520 N. Northwest Highway, Park Ridge, IL 60068-2573

[2] *Adapted from "Pain Control After Surgery: A Patient's Guide," February 1992, AHCPR Pub. No. 92-0021, Rockville, MD 20852.*
[3] *"Anesthesia & You . . . The Management of Pain," prepared by the American Society of Anesthesiologists through the cooperative efforts of the Society's Committee on Communications and the Committee on Pain Therapy, 1994.*

- "Pain Control After Surgery: A Patient's Guide," Agency for Health Care Policy and Research, Pub. No. 92-0021, Publications Clearing House, P.O. Box 8547, Silver Spring, MD 20907 or call 1-800-358-9295 or 301-495-3453. This booklet is also available in Spanish.

What Is a Certified Registered Nurse Anesthetist?

A Certified Registered Nurse Anesthetist (CRNA) is an individual who:

- Has earned a bachelor of science in nursing (BSN) or other appropriate baccalaureate degree.

- Has a license as a registered nurse.

- Has a minimum of one year of critical care nursing experience.

- Has completed a nurse anesthesia education program comprising twenty-four to thirty-six months of graduate work in both classroom and clinical experiences.

According to the American Association of Nurse Anesthetists, although some licensing laws regulating nurse anesthetists require CRNAs to work under the supervision or direction of a physician, no state requires that the physician need be an anesthesiologist. Similarly, the Joint Commission on Accreditation of Healthcare Organizations does not require that CRNAs be supervised by an anesthesiologist.

Today, "Certified Registered Nurse Anesthetists administer more than 65 percent of the 26 million anesthetics given to patients each year in the United States. In addition, CRNAs are the sole anesthesia providers in more than 70 percent of rural hospitals, allowing these medical facilities to provide obstetrical, surgical, and trauma stabilization services."[4]

SURGERY

When the day for your surgery arrives, you may feel a little anxious. This is perfectly normal. You have every reason to feel a little nervous. You are giving up control of your body to an operating team.

But if you have done your homework, you have checked out your surgeon's qualifications and are satisfied that he or she is an expert and can communicate properly with you before and after the surgery. You trust your surgeon and have shared your accurate medical history, information concerning surgeries, and concerns. You also have confidence in your anesthesiologist and have shared your medical information with him or her as well.

A nurse will come into your room and ask you to remove any dentures or partial dental bridges. This is no time for false modesty. Place them in the plastic cup provided so they don't get lost. Remove all jewelry and give it to a family member for safe keeping. The anesthesiologist will probably come in next to insert an IV into a vein in your hand or lower arm. At this time, a solution will drip into your vein. Later, before you leave your room for the OR, a medication to help you relax may be added into the IV line.

All that remains is for you to prepare yourself mentally. Positive attitudes do affect your body's chemistry and can help to intensify the healing process. Take a few deep breaths and slowly let them out. Visualize yourself enjoying a swift and uneventful recovery. Continue to do so when an orderly comes to transfer you to the gurney that will take you to the operating room. Ask for a pillow for your head if you need one.

---

[4] *"Access to Health Care," American Association of Nurse Anesthetists, Park Ridge, IL, 1996.*

Although you may have been told that your surgery is scheduled for a specific time, that doesn't mean when it actually begins.
Usually you are brought to a holding area first. There may be other
patients lined up in this area, waiting for their turn in one of the
operating rooms.

When you are moved into the operating room, you'll be transferred to the operating table, which is hard. Despite the bright
lights shining down on the table, you may be cold. If so, ask for an
extra blanket to keep you warm. It not only will keep you more
comfortable, but recent studies show that if you're warm, you will
experience less bleeding, have fewer infections, will heal faster, and
can be discharged from the hospital sooner than if you were chilly.
(Typically, operating rooms have been kept cool, around 65°F so
the surgeons wouldn't get overheated.) You'll see various people in
scrubs bustling around.

One of the nurses may ask you what surgery you are having.
It's not a joke or small talk. It's one more level of safeguard, even
though your chart will be double-checked. In some hospitals, the
circulating nurse reads aloud the type of surgery and, if applicable,
which side is being operated on, before the surgeon is permitted
to pick up a scalpel.

☞ Three tips if you decide to have elective surgery:

1. *Don't have surgery performed at a teaching hospital in
   July (because that's when the new residents arrive fresh
   out of medical school).*

2. *Don't have it scheduled for a Friday (because there's usually less staff around over the weekends).*

3. *Schedule it when you have additional help and more
   available time for recovery than suggested, as it often
   takes a little longer than the surgeons tell you to feel your
   old self again (or, perhaps, even better).*

You also may be asked what type of music you like, as many surgeons realize that even patients who are under a general anesthetic can hear and that music helps to relax them.

If you're having a regional or local anesthetic, you'll be aware that a sterile drape blocks your view of the operating field. That helps to prevent infection. The anesthesiologist will tell you just as he or she is about to put medication into the IV line to put you to sleep. The next thing you'll know, you'll be in the recovery room.

☞ There are several good free brochures you can send away for to help you learn more about an upcoming elective surgical procedure. They include:

- *"When You Need an Operation"*

    This is a series of four public information brochures which cover (1) "Who Should Do Your Operation?" (2) "What Will Your Operation Cost?" (3) "Giving Informed Consent" and (4) "Should You Seek Consultation (Second Opinion)?"

Write to the American College of Surgeons, 55 East Erie Street, Chicago, IL 60611.

- *"What You Should Know About Anesthesia"*

    American Society of Anesthesiologists, 520 North Northwest Highway, Park Ridge, IL 60068 or call (847) 825-5586 or the American Association of Nurse Anesthetists, 222 South Prospect Avenue, Park Ridge, IL 60068 or call (847) 692-7050.

CHAPTER 9

Orders: What Are They and Who Gives Them

In theory, it seems simple. The doctor gives an order involving patient care and the nursing staff carries it out. Although it sounds foolproof enough, in practice there is much room for error. Sometimes, as a health reporter in a renowned Boston medical center experienced, the mix-up in orders can be fatal.

WRITTEN ORDERS

Frequently the doctor's handwriting is actually so bad that the nursing staff and hospital pharmacist really cannot read it. "We usually get the blame when a mistake is made," a career registered nurse confided bitterly, "but the truth is that far too often we can't read what the doctor has written. There's no use trying to look over the notes on the chart and guessing what the order may be either. Even the notes are illegible."

It's not just the scrawl that is illegible. Numbers are sloppily made, decimal points omitted and/or misplaced, and abbreviations so carelessly crafted that they can easily be misread. One study notes that before filling almost 20 percent of medication orders, the hospital pharmacy must call the physician back to ask for a translation of what the poorly written order really said.

What can you, the patient, do to prevent errors in written orders? Write your own. That is, ask the physician what he or she is going to order for you and make your own notes. Then, if a nurse comes in with a particular medication, you'll know if it is the proper drug and in the exact dosage prescribed for you. Of course, unless you have your PDR (*Physician's Desk Reference*) at your bedside, you'll have no way of knowing if the physician prescribed the correct dosage for your weight and age, and with consideration for the other medications you're taking. Computer software programs come with checks and balances; shouldn't your medical care have a similar safety backup system?

VERBAL ORDERS

In their haste to conclude their hospital rounds so they can return to the office to see the staggering number of patients mandated by the HMOs, doctors may toss out verbal orders to the nurse as they are hurrying down the hall. Charge nurses interviewed for this book estimated that anywhere from 10 to 20 percent of the orders issued to their nursing staff were verbal and that frequently, physicians neglected to ever document and sign those orders on the patients' charts. If you've ever played the childhood game of telephone (where everyone sits in a circle and you repeat a message that the person on your left has whispered in your ear to the individual on your right), you'll know how quickly verbal messages can become distorted. Add to that confusion the similarity of names for many of today's pharmaceuticals along with a cacophony of both regional and foreign accents that can further distort the accuracy of the order, and you have a prescription for potential error.

Shortly after one woman's first baby was born, the infant developed a rash on her face. The pediatrician told her, so she thought, to buy the baby a net blanket. Like any good first-time mother, she raced from store to store, asking if each stocked this mysterious item. Finally, one rationally thinking salesclerk asked her who the pediatrician was. When she heard the name, she laughed. "Honey," she said, "he's a Southern boy. He was saying *knit* blanket."

While the above makes a good story, it wouldn't be so funny if it had been the wrong medication or dosage. Unfortunately, there isn't a great deal of control you as the patient can exert, other than to make the nursing staff more aware of possible errors by saying something like, "Dr. Jones sure has a thick accent. I hope he doesn't give verbal orders."

TELEPHONE ORDERS

Telephone orders also are ripe for misinterpretation. Static on the line or cell phone fade-out or interference may garble the message. Orders have to be signed by the physician and, of course, that is impossible over the phone, so the nurse is forced to carry out orders and then track the doctor down the next time he or she appears in person to sign what already has been done. Many physicians say that telephone orders are responsible for many malpractice suits because there is no verification and the case turns into a "He said" and "No, I didn't" argument.

As a patient, your only real defense against telephone orders is to ask the nurse what the doctor said (or what she or he *thought* the doctor said) and make note of it.

THE FIVE RULES OF DRUG ADMINISTRATION

You should always remain aware of the five rules of correct drug administration:

1. The right medication. Check your notes to make sure that the medication the physician said he or she was ordering for you is what you are being given. Remind the nurse of the other drugs you are taking to be sure that the present one is not contraindicated because of a possible harmful interaction.

2. The right dosage. Again, check your notes and verify the dosage originally indicated. The difference between 0.8 milligrams and 8.0 milligrams can be deadly. Also record in your own notebook the time you received your medication. If the nurse forgets to write on your chart that it was taken, another may think it was omitted and try to give you a second (and potentially harmful) dose.

3. The right patient. Be sure the nurse checks your identification bracelet. Always announce your complete name too, not just "I'm Mrs. Riley," but "I'm Jennifer Riley." Otherwise, the nurse may think she heard "Mrs. Wylie," nod, and give you Grace Wylie's injection. Do mistakes like that really happen? Unfortunately, yes.

4. The right route. Certain medications are supposed to be given by pill, liquid, or capsule, either orally or sublingually (under the tongue); others rectally; by transdermal patch; in an oral or nasal spray; intravenously (through an IV line); or intramuscularly (by injection or "IM" as it is called in medical jargon).

5. The right time. Dosages of most drugs are prescribed at specific times in order for the proper amount of the medication to remain in the body, not build up nor be absorbed too quickly. Often, however, due to an emergency situation with another patient or a shortage of staff on the floor, there may be a delay before the medicine actually is given. If pain builds up before more medication is given, it becomes much harder to control, which is why the PCA (patient-controlled analgesics) has become so popular with patients and nursing staff alike.

CHAPTER 10

How Families Can Help

I t's frightening to have a loved one in the hospital, especially when you've read this far in our book and know all the potential dangers lurking in bacteria-filled corners, on unwashed hands, and in mismarked medicines. Mix in your own personal concerns with the long-range effects of your family member's illness, fatigue factors, financial considerations, and the fear of possibly losing your loved one, and you're experiencing a high stress level.

Yet there are definite steps you can take to reassure yourself as well as your family member who's hospitalized and to reduce the tension and apprehension you both feel.

STAY CALM

There's never a good time for someone you love to be hospitalized. Everything may seem overwhelming as you mentally juggle car pools, child care, report deadlines, conferences, and speeches you'll have to reschedule with concerns about delayed or conflicting test results, questions about medical consultants, and fears of the unknown. You may feel as though your reasonable, predictable world has gone out of orbit and is zigzagging on a suicide course.[1]

Try not to panic. You *can* gain control of the situation and help protect your loved one who is in the hospital. The secret is

[1] *Adapted from Elaine Fantle Shimberg,* Strokes: What Families Should Know *(New York: Ballantine Books, 1990), 1.*

simple—learn as much as you can as quickly as you can and ask questions freely. As the Chinese philosopher Confucius said, "The essence of knowledge is, having it, to apply it; not having it, to confess your ignorance."

KNOW THE PLAYERS

The key to any situation is to know where the power lies. You can gain this information by rereading Chapter 3 and knowing who the players are. You'll save time and patience, for example, by learning the name of the charge nurse on your loved one's floor or ward. This is the person who can quickly give you information about the patient's condition, change of medication, or treatment procedures. He or she is the captain of the team, so go to the top. If you don't receive satisfaction here, ask to speak with the patient advocate or hospital administrator.

Do not lose your temper, become rude, or use sarcasm when you're talking to the charge nurse or hospital administrator. You and your loved one need their understanding and cooperation. Remind yourself that you're under a tremendous emotional strain and, if it helps, utilize visualization, deep breathing, and self-talk to help you maintain control. Although hospital staff may understand that you're frightened, angry, concerned, frustrated, and exhausted, you still do, as your mother told you, get more flies with honey than vinegar.

LEARN ABOUT THE HOSPITAL STAFF AND POLICIES

The quickest way to learn all you can about the hospital staff and policies is to read all the materials handed out to you at admissions. Most of us just blindly stuff those brochures into a purse or briefcase and forget about them. But the hospital's public relations department spent a great deal of time (and money) preparing these materials because they thought they were important; and they probably are. Skim over the "puff pieces" and focus—underline or highlight so you can retrieve the information quickly—on the material that affects you or your hospitalized family member.

Usually, these brochures tell you the name of the patient advocate, a staff member assigned to handle problems experienced by patients or their families. It pays to learn that name and, if possible, to seek that individual out to introduce yourself even before there are any problems. It makes you and your family member "real people," rather than the cardiac patient in room 602.

It also doesn't hurt to be friendly with the nursing staff. Many families bring candy, cookies, bagels, or a fruit basket to leave at the nurses' station, with a card saying "From the (their name) Family." It's not a bribe, just common courtesy to thank these tireless men and women who have direct influence over the care your family member will receive. Bring it shortly after your family member has been admitted, rather than waiting until you leave. (You also can send a "thank you" basket after your loved one is home safely as well.)

Be considerate of the hospital staff's time and energy. They are there to help the patients, not the patients' families. Don't ask them to furnish soap and towels so you can shower or to help you make up your "bed" for the night. While they are probably grateful that you are staying full time to help with the patient (which does ease their work load considerably), they also are aware that they will be tripping over you every time they come into the room and that you will be watching their every move, which is why you are staying in the first place.

Be friendly and courteous. Ask questions if you need to, but don't stop the nurses for idle chatter. They have other patients to care for, patients who probably don't have anyone watching out for them.

Make yourself useful: Fill the water pitcher (ask first if it's permitted), help the patient at mealtime, answer the phone when it's hard for the patient to reach, and move the flowers out of the way so they don't get knocked over. But know your limits. Don't try to get your family member out of bed unless you know how to support him or her to prevent dangerous falls. Never touch the IV line, dressings, catheter, or other invasive tubing. Instead, call for the nurse.

LEARN ALL YOU CAN ABOUT YOUR FAMILY MEMBER'S ILLNESS

Many hospitals have medical libraries where family members can read up on a particular illness or treatment. Ask about these facilities as the hospital staff may not mention them. Remember, however, that there usually is at least an 18-month period between the time a book is written, published, and sold to the public. Technology—especially in the medical field—often changes overnight. Any book you are reading—even one just published—may contain dated information. Although magazines and journals have shorter lead time between writing, submission, and publication, it may be as much as nine months, so they also could present some obsolete information.

If you're comfortable with computers and have a modem, you can gain additional information about new technology and treatment procedures as well as names of experts in a particular field by accessing the Internet and medical data banks like Med Line. Don't forget the special interest bulletin boards and chat lines on America Online, Prodigy, and CompuServe where you can "talk" with others facing similar medical problems. Often, family members have become aware of advances or new procedures in a particular medical area before their physician has read about it in the journals.

If you have no idea how to turn on a computer, let alone find the World Wide Web, call your nearest high school or the business school of a local college and ask for the names of students you could hire to help you.

While you may hear about some new or experimental treatment from family members, friends, or computer chat lines, remember that every illness is unique to the individual who has it; what helped your neighbor's mother may not be beneficial to yours.

BECOME THE PATIENT'S EYES AND EARS

You know the patient better than anyone, certainly better than the doctors and nurses. You may notice subtle changes in behavior before they do. Make notes of anything that seems changed and alert the medical staff immediately. For example, you may notice that your elderly father seems a little confused and is having trouble forming his words. The nursing staff may assume he's just old and that this is normal for him. You, on the other hand, know that he just won the chess championship in the over-eighty division at his club and that he is the oldest member of the local Toastmaster's Club. His confusion and slight aphasia (partial loss in the ability to use or understand words) could be due to a transient ischemic attack (TIA, otherwise known as a "little stroke") or a problem with his various medications.

You also need to keep a list of all medications your family member is being given, how they are administered, when, and at what dosage. Know what these drugs look like as well. The library has a book called *Physician's Desk Reference* (PDR) that describes the dosages and potential side effects of drugs and has colored pictures illustrating what they look like.

Also, keep a list of any known allergies or other medical conditions. Many caregivers put this information in a loose-leaf notebook with dividers, so the material can be quickly accessed when needed. This notebook stays in the room with the patient until he or she is discharged. Keeping all the information in one place also makes it easier for a respite replacement to take over if you have to leave briefly. Be sure to have extra notepaper so additional material can be added.

If your family member is visually or hearing impaired, be sure that fact is posted over the bed so anyone—a physician, nurse, aide, or technician—is aware. Otherwise, someone might enter the room and touch the patient, assuming that he or she knew the person was in the room. A patient who is hearing impaired could miss valuable instructions that might affect his or her medical care. Be sure this information is also marked conspicuously on your family member's chart, in case he or she is taken out of the room for tests or surgery.

REASSURE AND REORIENT YOUR FAMILY MEMBER

Studies confirm that patients who are more relaxed tend to feel less pain, heal more quickly, and experience less depression than those who are fearful or overly concerned about their condition. Your reassurance can help strengthen your family member's power of the mind to heal the body.

Don't stand in the room and whisper, even if you think the patient is sleeping or still unconscious. Research tells us that patients can hear what is being said, even while they're under anesthetic. Even if you're only whispering about baseball scores, your family member may think you know something about his or her medical condition and fear the worst. The thought always is, "Perhaps they're not telling me everything."

Many family members and friends come to visit a patient, then talk to each other, ignoring the one who is ill. It can be exhausting to a patient who probably is not sleeping too well as it is. Try to limit the number of visitors. If you can't, then limit the visiting time period. Blame it on the nursing staff if you have to. They won't mind.

Don't feel you have to talk constantly when you are with your loved one. Sometimes just sitting quietly, holding hands, speaks volumes.

Help reorient the patient to the present surroundings, especially if it's someone who is elderly. With the activity and noise level found on the typical hospital floor, it's easy to become confused as to location and lose track of time. If there's no clock or calendar in the room, bring them from home.

Bring an extra family photo in an inexpensive frame (it might disappear if it's an expensive frame) to help comfort the patient. It also will remind technicians, nurses, and doctors coming along bedside that this is not just Mrs. Anderson in room 303 with recurring stomach cancer, but a human being who also has a husband, three adult children, and a new grandson. It helps to humanize and personalize the person in the bed.

As patients often are transferred from one floor to another for various reasons, you also may need to remind your family member of the room number, floor or ward, and sometimes even which hospital he or she is in. This is particularly important if your family member has had frequent recent hospitalizations.

Let your hospitalized family member know what has happened to him or her, emphasizing what is normal and expected under the circumstances. If someone has suffered a stroke, for example, say, "You've had a stroke. Right now you can't move your left arm." Even if the patient can't speak, it's reassuring to know what has transpired.

One stroke survivor admitted, "I thought I was going crazy. They asked me questions and I answered. Then they asked me again. Finally, my daughter said, 'Daddy, I know *you* know what you're saying, but you're not making the right words. We can't understand you.' Thank God she told me. It made me feel better to understand why nobody seemed to be listening to me."

TOUCH

Don't be afraid to touch your hospitalized loved one. Our skin is the largest and most sensitive organ in our body. Yet, when family members are sickest, we often hesitate to reach out to comfort them by a gentle stroke or caress. Perhaps it is a fear of dislodging the various tubes and monitors or of causing additional pain.

Yet, studies have shown that a reassuring pat can speed recovery and that touch is a most-needed nurturing ingredient for all human beings, from birth throughout the aging process. Petting a dog or cat actually lowers blood pressure, which is one of the reasons that pet therapy has been introduced to nursing homes as well as pediatric and general hospitals. The "laying on of hands" has calmed and cured many when medical technology could not.

The late Norman Cousins, writing about his own physical illness and hospitalization in *Anatomy of an Illness,* describes the "... utter void created by the longing—ineradicable, unremitting, pervasive—for warmth of human contact. A warm smile and an outstretched hand were valued even above the offerings of modern science, but the latter were far more accessible than the former."[2]

MAINTAIN YOUR SENSE OF HUMOR

In *Anatomy of an Illness,* Norman Cousins also described in detail how he felt the power of laughter helped to cure him of a painful and crippling disease. Numerous studies support the importance of laughter, saying that it stimulates the brain to release powerful chemical agents called endorphins that help to reduce pain. Hearty laughter, the kind we call belly laughter, causes you to breathe deeply, bringing in more oxygen to your lungs. Researchers at many medical centers have found that laughter also boosts the immune system.

Although laughter has recently been encouraged for its healing properties by physicians-authors Bernie Siegel, M.D., and Deepak Chopra, M.D., to name just two, the idea is nothing new. Proverbs 17:22 says, "A merry heart doeth good like a medicine." Since 1930, *Reader's Digest* has printed its popular column "Laughter, the Best Medicine." And Charlie Chaplin, known to the world as silent film's "funniest man," once said, "Laughter is the tonic, the relief, the surcease for pain."

Recognizing the power of laughter, many hospitals now include comedy videotapes and stand-up comic audiotapes in

[2]Norman Cousins, *Anatomy of an Illness* (New York: Bantam Books, 1981), 154.

their libraries for patient use in their rooms, as well as collections of humor and joke books. Follow their example and encourage friends and family members to bring humor, not long faces, into the hospital room when they visit.

MAKE TIME FOR YOURSELF

It's easy to feel schizophrenic when you have a loved one in the hospital. You want to be with him or her—and you or someone always should be, but it doesn't have to be *just* you. You may also have other responsibilities—children, elderly parents, business, and so on, so you feel torn, frustrated, and exhausted. Sometimes your car pulls into the hospital parking lot without your even remembering how you got there.

Yet your first concern must always be to protect yourself. Only then you can help your hospitalized family member. If you recall, airlines always tell their passengers that when the oxygen masks fall during an emergency, first put the mask on yourself, then on a small child or infant.

Dr. Peter Dunne, a Tampa neurologist, tells of a woman who never left her sick husband's side while he was in the hospital. "He had suffered a major stroke," Dr. Dunne related, "and although he was very ill, I felt he had a good chance for a reasonable recovery. I urged the woman to go home to get some rest, to eat properly, to care for herself. She ignored my pleading. She wore herself out. Ironically, she suffered a heart attack and died. There was no one else to care for her husband, and he had to be sent to a nursing home. If only she had kept her priorities straight."[3]

What could this woman have done to give herself some respite? She was the only relative her husband had. But she lived in a world with others who could have helped her and become her support system if only they had known she needed help. Many

[3] *Elaine Fantle Shimberg,* Depression: What Families Should Know *(New York: Ballantine Books, 1991), 121.*

churches and synagogues have volunteers who are willing to spend some scheduled time with those who are ill—in the hospital or at home—so the caregiver can have some time off. (If yours doesn't, get involved with organizing such a program.) Other community groups also provide respite care. Most hospitals have social workers who are aware of each particular community's services. But unless you ask for help, you may not receive it. Do not become a martyr. They're all dead.

CHAPTER 11

How to Heal Faster

With the acknowledgment that hospitals are not the healthiest places to be, the goal should be to heal quickly and get discharged from the hospital as soon as possible. (The insurance company's goal, of course, is merely to get you discharged from the hospital as quickly as possible.)

If you've read this far in our book, you know we feel strongly that becoming a patient does not and should not mean assuming a state of passivity. There is much you as a patient can and should do to improve your well-being while you are hospitalized.

YOUR BODY'S ABILITY TO HEAL ITSELF

One much needed contribution is to understand, intensify, and utilize your body's ability to heal itself. There is nothing New Age or magical about it. An increasing number of doctors and major hospitals already acknowledge the belief in the interaction of mind and body. According to an article in the June 24, 1996 issue of *Time* magazine, "more and more medical schools are adding courses on holistic and alternative medicine with titles like 'Caring for the Soul.'" Dr. Herbert Benson, associate professor of medicine at Harvard Medical Institute, director of the Mind/Body Medical Institute, coauthor of *The Relaxation Response* and *Timeless Healing,* and author of *The Mind/Body Effect,* says "Scientific studies demonstrate that by repeating prayers, words or sounds, and passively disregarding other thoughts, many people are able to trigger a specific set of physiological changes including decreased metabolism, heart rate, rate of breathing, and distinctive, slower brain waves."

A panel of the National Institutes of Health, composed of twelve experts in behavior, pain and sleep medicines, nursing, psychology, and neurology, concluded that meditation, hypnosis, relaxation, and biofeedback were valid alternative treatments to be used in combination with conventional treatments. According to the panel, "Available data support the effectiveness of these interventions in relieving chronic pain and in achieving some reduction in insomnia." They admitted that the particular approach could vary according to the individual patient.

Surgeon and author Bernie Siegel writes in his numerous books of patients who were able to use their mental powers to help control bleeding during and after surgeries. In her book, *Imagery in Healing,* psychologist Jeanne Achterberg cites studies supporting the impact of the imagination on such physiological processes as salivation, heart rate, muscle tension, gastrointestinal activity, blister formation, blood pressure, and respiration. The late Norman Cousins, author of *Anatomy of an Illness* and *The Healing Heart,* emphasized that "positive attitudes and emotions can affect the biochemistry of the body to facilitate rejuvenation and health." Women choosing to deliver their babies by natural childbirth methods have learned to incorporate relaxation techniques, visualization, and self-hypnosis to control the pain of childbirth. Yoga, Tai Chi, poetry, and some types of music can also stimulate relaxation.

There are numerous books and tapes that can help you learn to relax, visualize, or use self-hypnosis to boost your immune system and to reduce pain. They include (but are not limited to) *The Relaxation Response* by Herbert Benson, M.D., with Miriam Z. Klipper; *How to Meditate* by Lawrence LeShan; *Minding the Body, Mending the Mind* by Joan Borysenko; *The New Physics of Healing* and *Quantum Healing* by Deepak Chopra, M.D.; and *Positive Imaging: The Powerful Way to Change Your Life* by Norman Vincent

Peale. So many world-renowned authors, all with the same message: The power to heal our body comes from within us.

It takes practice, though, so don't expect success the first time you try. You may feel somewhat self-conscious the first time you try relaxation exercises, meditation, or visualization. It sounds so . . . well, New Age. But once you've read some of the books by qualified physicians, men and women with outstanding credentials from the world's top medical institutions, you'll begin to open your mind to new ideas. Read the supportive research written up in prestigious medical journals. Talk to others who have used self-hypnosis or visualization to reduce pain and anxiety from minor medical and dental procedures, to boost their immunity, and to recover quickly from surgery.

Like a child cautiously dipping a toe in the cold water of the ocean, you'll venture forth. Success. We can both vouch for the joy (and relief) and the sense of wonderment that envelops you when you discover how simple it is, how natural. Your mind *does* affect your body. These are not two separate entities. They are one, forever intertwined, functioning as they were meant to, if only you permit this magic to occur. In his book, *Quantum Healing,* Dr. Deepak Chopra states, ". . . a level of total, deep relaxation is the most important precondition for curing any disorder. The underlying concept is that the body knows how to maintain balance unless thrown off by disease; therefore if one wants to restore the body's own healing ability, everything should be done to bring it back to balance."[1]

If you try one audiotape and it doesn't help you achieve the restful state you desire, try another. Some people react better to the sound of a male voice than a female, or vice versa. There may be music on the tape that distracts you, rather than helping you to reach the alpha state of brain activity. "One size" doesn't fit all in this situation. Keep searching until you find the right tape for you.

[1] *Deepak Chopra, M.D.,* Quantum Healing *(New York: Bantam Books, 1989), 14.*

You might be more successful by making your own tape, including your choice of music to help you focus. Some people prefer no music at all. Many of the above-mentioned books include sample scripts that you can adapt to your own needs and read into a tape recorder.

Patients often take these relaxation tapes with them to the hospital. Besides providing pleasure and relaxation, they help to drown out the frightening sounds of the beeping heart monitor, moans and groans from other patients, and the banter between the nurses. Use them during painful or uncomfortable procedures or during surgery itself. Be sure to tell your surgeon and anesthesiologist that you are doing so. Believe in your power to help your body heal itself. Millions of others do.

In his book, *Peace, Love & Healing,* surgeon Bernie Siegel writes, "I expect hospitals will in the future use closed-circuit television in patients' rooms to provide preoperative preparation, meditation, healing imagery, music and laughter. Sooner or later they'll see that this will help patients heal faster, and reduce hospitalization costs. Wellness is cost-effective."[2] Dr. Siegel, like many other surgeons, uses music in the operating room, believing that the patients can hear the music and relax, even though they are under a general anesthetic.

MUSIC SOOTHES, THEREBY PROMOTING HEALING

In 1697, English playwright William Congreve wrote, "Music hath charms to soothe a savage breast, To soften rocks, or bend a knotted oak." Music has far more than charms, it seems. It also possesses great therapeutic powers.

Music therapy is hardly a modern technique. The Bible tells of King David's playing on his harp to cure Saul of his depression. Ancient physicians used singing and crude musical instruments to

---

[2]*Bernie Siegel, M.D.*, Peace, Love & Healing *(New York: Harper & Row, 1989), 143.*

bring a rapid heartbeat under control and to otherwise comfort their patients. Even today, medicine men and healers in many cultures use singing and chanting to help heal their patients.

Scientific studies have shown the positive effect music can have on pain control. Even anesthetized patients undergoing surgery while music is being played reportedly require less pain medication during their recovery. The reason for this is that music—both its sound and vibrations—releases endorphins, powerful chemicals produced in the brain that help to relieve pain and trigger relaxation. Music affects our body's respiration rate, blood pressure, heartbeat, and hormonal level. In fact, many hospitals now use music in their intensive coronary care units to help control blood pressure in their coronary patients. Relaxing music also reduces stress levels and can actually help to speed up the healing process. It also can reduce depression, which often is present after surgery or a serious illness.

Particular songs can stir up memories of happier (and healthier) times, triggering what Dr. Herbert Benson refers to as "remembered wellness." Neurologist Oliver Sacks, author of *Awakenings*, *An Anthropologist on Mars, The Man Who Mistook His Wife for a Hat*, and *A Leg to Stand On*, described in an article in a 1991 issue of the *Journal of the American Medical Association* (JAMA) how music triggered key memories in patients who had lost their ability to retrieve past associations. In Dr. Sacks' book *An Anthropologist on Mars* he describes a musicologist who was ". . . unable to remember events or facts for more than a few seconds, but able to remember, and indeed to learn, elaborate musical pieces, to conduct them, to perform them, and even to improvise at the organ."[3] Music also has been used successfully in treating patients with Parkinson's disease and is being tried with those suffering from Alzheimer's disease. Over sixty colleges and universities in the United States now offer a degree in music therapy as a treatment modality.

---

[3] Oliver Sacks, An Anthropologist on Mars *(New York: Alfred A. Knopf, 1995)*, 65.

Ask a family member to bring you a small radio or soothing instrumental music cassettes to help you relax and heal faster. Select music with the tempo akin to your heartbeat, between seventy and eighty times a minutes. Even humming can help you to relax, slow your heartbeat, and feel less pain and discomfort. Practice progressive relaxation while focusing on your favorite music. Chances are you'll quickly slip into the alpha wave state which is one of total relaxation. If not, however, don't get discouraged. Stop trying so hard; it will eventually happen. Just permit tension and anxiety to be carried away on the fading strains of each note.

PRACTICE YOUR BREATHING

After surgery you may be visited by a respiratory therapist who will tell you to practice your deep breathing. Often, that's the last thing you want to do because it hurts. That's why you're taking shallow breaths—because it's far less painful.

But the therapist isn't being sadistic, although you may think so at the time. What the medical staff often forgets to tell you is that after you have had anesthesia, traces of the various drugs used to numb your body still remain in your lungs. Baby breaths don't fill your lungs with enough oxygen to rid your body of these medications. There also may be mucus plugs that have collected in your bronchial tubes that need to be coughed up so you don't develop pneumonia.

Hug that pillow or teddy bear they give you to support your chest or stomach incision and breathe deeply as instructed. Don't go too fast and rest between inhalations so you don't hyperventilate. Although you may be on the honor system to do these exercises, don't be tempted to cheat and not do them exactly as advised. You're the one who will pay, and painfully.

A technician or nurse may bring a breathing device (called an incentive spirometer) into your room and instruct you to blow into the mouthpiece, which is attached to tubing leading to a

☞ Never practice coughing unless instructed by the nurse or respiratory therapist. There are certain medical conditions, such as eye injuries or eye surgery, where coughing could be detrimental.

see-through plastic container with a ball inside. Your job will be to blow hard enough into the mouthpiece to make the ball jump. (It also encourages you to take a deep breath before you blow.) The purpose of this exercise is to help you clear your lungs. Before you begin, however, ask how the equipment is sterilized. It may be a disposable mouthpiece and tubing, but until you are satisfied that you are breathing into a bacteria-free mouthpiece and tubing, refuse to participate until a supervisor can convince you of its safety.

MINIMIZE PAIN

Pain control is important because the body is more able to heal itself when relatively pain free. Patients also are more relaxed and able to perform physical therapy when pain is minimized. Yet studies show a high prevalence of needless unrelieved pain among hospitalized patients. A major reason for this is that few physicians are trained in medical school to understand the healing benefits derived from the alleviation of pain or the importance of asking patients about their pain level. Nurses as a group tend to be more aware of their patients' discomfort because they interact more with their patients. Yet research reveals that complaints of pain are seldom charted on a patient's record.

Traditionally, certain groups of patients, such as children, the elderly, people in the ICU, and non–English-speaking patients, are not given adequate pain medication, because it is difficult to communicate with them to ascertain how much pain they are experiencing. Older patients tend to be stoic about their pain, preferring to bear it in silence rather than "making waves" and possibly upsetting the nursing staff. Until recently, it was thought that children did not experience pain in the same way adults did, so they were given far less analgesia than they actually required. Often children hesitate to report pain because they don't want to be considered a baby or are afraid of being given an injection, not understanding that the immediate discomfort from the needle would relieve their overall pain.

Many patients reject medication to control their pain because they are worried about becoming addicted. While this may be a concern in long-term cases, it rarely occurs when used short-term. Unfortunately, however, some physicians also subscribe to this type of thinking, and underprescribe pain medication for their patients.

But don't wait for your doctor to ask if you are experiencing any "discomfort." Speak up. Describe your pain and its intensity. Many hospitals use a zero to ten rating, with zero being no pain at all and ten being excruciating pain. If the patient is your child, see if the hospital has pictorial pain charts with sketches of smiling faces and frowning ones. Ask your youngster to point at the one that shows how much he or she is hurting. Then be sure that this evaluation is placed on the chart.

Discuss your concerns about pain with your physician, nurse, or anesthesiologist. Don't try to be stoic or think it's macho to bear the pain. There's no need to suffer. There are many analgesics available today that can help to minimize pain.

Many physicians today use patient-controlled analgesics (PCA) in which the patient is able to control the frequency of the pain medication by pushing a button to release a controlled dosage. Patient-controlled analgesics are safe, thanks to numerous mechanical safeguards, and have proven so successful that this technique is used with selected patients in many children's hospitals, including the world-renowned Shriners Hospitals. According to anesthesiologists interviewed for this book, patients using PCA actually use less pain medication because they are able to control its delivery by need.

> Often, nurses will hand you a pill or appear with a syringe and say, "Here's something for your pain." Although you feel relieved, remember to first ask, "What is it?" Always know the name of the medication you're receiving. It could be something to which you have a known allergy, about to be given to you by mistake.

Additional benefits, according to an article in the November/December 1990 issue of *Pediatric Nursing,* include "...earlier, more comfortable postoperative ambulation, more immediate relief of pain with less sedation, fewer postoperative pulmonary complications, and improved cooperation with postoperative physical therapy." It also frees the nursing staff to spend more time caring for their patients.

Don't expect the medical staff to read your mind if you're in pain or, unfortunately, to even ask you about your pain. Speak up. If the patient is an elderly family member, you may have to have to read between the lines to determine how much discomfort there is. Some of the behavioral cues include restlessness, such as tossing their head from side to side or rocking; sighing or moaning; sad or frightened facial expression; crying; or obvious body tension.

There are additional ways to control pain, other than with drugs. Sometimes they are used in combination with analgesics. These nonpharmaceutical methods include visualization, relaxation techniques, distraction, biofeedback, and self-hypnosis.

LEARN THE LINGO

It's important for you to learn the medical lingo because answers you give to questions asked may have a direct bearing on follow-up treatment and could help or hinder your healing process.

For example, the nurse may tell you she's put a "cap" in the bathroom in order to "measure your urinary output." What she means is that she has put a plastic insert under the toilet seat so she can see how much you've peed.

You may be asked if you have a "productive" cough. Translated, it means, are you coughing up mucus?

If asked if you were bleeding profusely (or had prolonged bleeding) before entering the hospital, find out what the questioner means by "profusely" (or prolonged). Some medical professionals may help to qualify their questions by saying, "Would you say there was a tablespoon of blood? A cup?" or even "Did you bleed continuously for five minutes? Ten? Half an hour?" Others, however, never consider that their definition of "heavy bleeding" could be different from yours. The result could be hazardous to your recovery as vague language can channel you into an erroneous treatment modality.

If you don't understand what the nurse, physician, or technician is asking you, speak up. Tell them to please rephrase the question so you can fully understand it.

NEVER UNDERESTIMATE THE POWER OF PRAYER

Dr. Bernie S. Siegel writes in his books that spiritual people have a higher recovery rate. "They refuse to see themselves as victims," he says. ". . . They also call on God. True peace of mind comes when you have a divine source to help, support, and accompany you, to get you through difficulties and to show you the strength you really have. A relationship with God can help you overcome things that defeat other people."[4]

Pediatric neurosurgeon Fred Epstein, M.D., formerly of New York University Medical Center and presently Chairman of the

---

[4]*From an interview with Aron Hirt-Manheimer, "Overcoming Our Pain: The Life Lessons of Dr. Bernie S. Siegel,"* Reform Judaism *24, no. 4 (Summer 1996): 42.*

Department of Neurosurgery and Director of the Institute for Neurology and Neurosurgery at Beth Israel Hospital in New York City, operates on tumors in kids' brains and on spinal cords that other neurosurgeons call "inoperable." Says Epstein, "People often ask me if I'm a believer. I always answer, 'In this business, you have to be.' I know that we are in the hands of a higher power, especially at the moment of greatest risk."

Numerous physicians have echoed this thought, adding that there are no atheists in the operating room. The power of prayer, long expressed by clergy and laypeople alike, is now being acknowledged by the medical community as well. Researcher Dale Matthews of Georgetown University studied 212 medical cases and found that "Three-fourths showed a positive effect of religious commitment on health." This research also shows benefits of religion on dealing with drug abuse, alcoholism, depression, cancer, high blood pressure, and heart disease.

Tampa surgeon Sylvia Campbell says she's always paid attention to her patients' spiritual needs as well as their physical and emotional needs. "I never force a conversation about prayer on my patients," she stressed. "I'll open the door and if someone walks through it, I'm there for them. There's no science to prayer," she adds. "It's a matter of faith. You either have it or you don't. Faith is like the wind. You don't see it or taste it, but you can feel it. You know it's there."

Harold Koenig of Duke University Medical Center cited a study now in progress of 4,000 elderly women. Preliminary results show "people who attend church are both physically healthier and less depressed."

Former Surgeon General C. Everett Koop said, "I expect to see more research on the effect of prayer in the healing process. People will start talking a lot more, not just about mental attitudes on their bodies, but the attitude of spirituality. Doctors . . . if they're smart, use whatever the patient has to help that patient's healing."

Some experts, like Herbert Benson, say taking part in prayer may lower harmful stress hormones, such as adrenaline, in the body. Reducing this kind of stress level can reduce high blood pressure, chronic pain, insomnia, and anxiety, thereby helping the body to heal more efficiently.

Sometimes it doesn't even matter who does the praying; in 1988, a study of 393 patients in a California coronary care unit revealed that the group being prayed for by others suffered fewer episodes of congestive heart failure or cardiac arrest, had less incidence of pneumonia, and required less medication than those receiving no regular organized prayers. Interestingly, neither group knew whether they were or were not being prayed for.

A quarter of U.S. medical schools now offer courses that address spirituality. In 1995, Harvard Medical School sponsored a three-day conference on the subject of health care and spirituality. It was attended by almost 1000 scientists, physicians, psychologists, sociologists, and theologians.

What does all this talk about spirituality have to do with you? It suggests that you might try opening your heart to the power of prayer even if you haven't tried it since your parents dragged you to religious school. Many hospitals have pastoral care volunteers, both ordained clergy and laity. Even if the individual is not of your religious faith, he or she may be able to guide you in prayer. Sometimes it isn't as much what is said, as that you are asking for help to find the strength within yourself.

ENCOURAGE THE HEALING TOUCH

Many children's hospitals and nursing homes encourage "pet therapy," in which animals—usually dogs—are brought into the facility to be petted and hugged by the patients. Unfortunately, most adult hospitals don't permit pets, personal or otherwise, to visit. Yet research shows that stroking a pet and being on the receiving end of a pet's loving licks can lower blood pressure and have other positive effects on one's health.

One woman learned the value of pet therapy firsthand after her elderly father had suffered a series of debilitating strokes. After one particularly serious stroke, he seemed to slip into a coma and for two weeks was unresponsive to any type of stimuli. On one visit, she and her daughter smuggled in one of the daughter's new kittens.

"I put the kitten on my father's chest," she recalled. "His frail hands were folded over his chest and slowly moved up and down with his breathing. The kitten looked around, blinked, then sat down on Daddy's chest and began licking his hands with her rough little tongue. Slowly, my father's eyes opened. He looked down at the kitten, then smiled. 'Now that's what I call a kitten,' he said. These were the first words he had said in weeks."

Often, when we're in the hospital, we don't feel or look our best. It's easy to retreat from friends and family, to become depressed and withdrawn. Be on guard for these negative emotions and don't allow them to happen to you or a hospitalized loved one. Reach out to those who can comfort you; encourage your children and grandchildren to visit. Ask "fun friends," those buddies who make you laugh and feel good, to come to see you as well. They may hesitate, not wanting to bother you while you're in the hospital. But these special healers are important to your well-being. Their tender touches are more than merely soothing; they can have a profound positive impact on the immune system and other bodily functions.

By the same token, if you have friends, acquaintances, or even family members who give off negative energy and make you feel anxious or depressed, ask them to stay home. Their depression can be contagious. Promise them (with your fingers crossed) that they can visit you at home when you're feeling better (and are physically and emotionally stronger to cope with them). Blame it on this book, if you need to.

Recently, enlightened medical professionals have taken a page from the writings of most of the major religions of the world and are realizing the benefits of "the laying on of hands." It has long been acknowledged that newborn infants and geriatric patients alike fare far better when they are tactilely stimulated. There actually is a potentially fatal wasting disease called marasmus that affects new-borns who are not properly stimulated. An article in the January/February 1996 issue of *American Health* described a study at the University of Miami Touch Research Institute in which researchers found that "premature babies who got three 15-minute massages a day had a 47 percent greater weight gain and shorter hospital stays than preemies who didn't."[5]

Hospitalized patients also benefit from the positive strokes from massage. In addition, studies now show that surgical patients fortunate enough to be cared for by nurses trained in the practice of "therapeutic touch" techniques tend to suffer less depression and less post-operative pain, thus requiring less medication and preventing the unwanted side effects that accompany many analgesics.

"Therapeutic touch," a technique that was developed in the early 1970s at the New York University Division of Nursing by Dolores Krieger, Ph.D., R.N., presently is used by thousands of nurses throughout the world. The treatment is recognized by the College of Nurses of Ontario (CNO) and is actively promoted by the Canadian Holistic Nurses Association. According to Roger Goodman, Director of Communications of the CNO, "Therapeutic touching is one of many 'complementary therapies' along with acupressure, visualization, and imagery." It has strong spiritual overtones.

In therapeutic touch, the practitioner does not actually touch the patient's body. (Touching that does involve physical contact falls more into the realm of massage, which also can be beneficial.) Instead, his or her hands are held a few inches from the patient's skin, moving them along the body, tapping into a "universal energy force" and transferring some of it to the patient. The patient's hemoglobin level actually tends to rise, bringing with it increased oxygen levels throughout the body. While this may sound extremely New Age, one nurse trained in the procedure says, "It's

---

[5]Daryn Eller, "*Rubbed the Right Way*," American Health (January/February 1996): 75.

really a return to what nurses used to do. We've gone back to comforting and caring."

Therapeutic touch is used in neonatal intensive-care units along with actual touching, stroking, and gently patting the infant. It's also proven very successful in working with geriatric patients, as well as with any patient willing to accept actual physical comforting through touch. As with all therapies, said Goodman, therapeutic touch should be done only with the patients' informed consent. "Patients must accept the partnership role," Goodman stressed. "They must become involved not only in the total care plan, but also in the process of ongoing assessment as to the benefit of the particular plan."

Although therapeutic touch neither cures patients nor replaces standard medical protocols, it does help patients to relax and energize their body's immune system. Healing rates may actually increase after therapeutic touch is used. An article by Joan Breckenridge published in *The Toronto Globe and Mail* highlighted one of the best studies on therapeutic touch.[6] It was a randomized, double-blind experiment in which forty-four men with identical surgical biopsies on their arms were asked to put their arms through an opening in a wall. Twenty-three of the men received therapeutic touch; the others didn't. Slightly over two weeks later, the wound site on thirteen of those receiving therapeutic touch were completely healed, while none in the untreated group were fully healed. Many other studies are now being conducted in the United States.

Don't ever hesitate to ask for someone to hold your hand, soothe your brow, or gently rub your feet. Family and friends may feel shy about offering, but may be more than willing to oblige. Ask if any of the nursing staff is trained in therapeutic touch, although many who are don't advertise the fact. Nevertheless, touching can be strong medicine and play an important part in your healing. Reach out for it.

---

[6]Joan Breckenridge, *"Hands-off Treatment Moves In,"* The Toronto Globe and Mail, *9 July 1994, A1, A11.*

CHAPTER 12

Your Insurance Can Be Hazardous to Your Health

As we write this, we jointly muse that the practice of medicine today reminds us somewhat of the child's game of musical chairs: Everyone is scrambling to find a chair before the music stops. And you know who's left standing: the patient.

Hospitals are forging new partnerships—with medical practices, with other hospitals, and with other health agencies. This latter merger, called an integrated care delivery system, purportedly offers patients greater continuity between hospital and home health care or hospice services. It also limits choices for the patient. The old expression, "You pays your money, you gets your choice," doesn't seem to be applicable anymore, at least not when it comes to health insurance.

Often, your particular health care insurance dictates where you will receive your medical care and by whom. If you're lucky, that may be a board-certified competent and understanding physician and at a convenient hospital with a record for high quality and experience in caring for your particular medical problem, low mortality rates, and minimal infection rates. Obviously, the more procedures done by a physician in a particular hospital, the more the team becomes experienced as well as prepared for the unexpected to occur.

On the other hand, studies show that particular areas of the country as well as specific hospitals within a community often are more likely to perform operations that may be unnecessary—such as tonsillectomies, hysterectomies, and cesareans—than others. If you're assigned to a particular physician's group or hospital where the standard of care mandates surgery rather than more conservative treatment, demand a second opinion.

WHO BENEFITS FROM INSURANCE?

We've come a long way since the old family doctor was paid in chickens or a side of beef when money for payment was in short supply. Since the early 1970s, a baffling array of insurance plans has sprung up, mutating coverage until few can really comprehend what services are or are not covered and under which circumstances. Today there are approximately 600 health maintenance organizations (HMOs) in the United States, insuring more than 50 million people with another 70 million subscribers in other types of health-care plans. Most medical offices have hired additional staff just to handle insurance claims and to spend the necessary hours on the telephone trying to get authorization for tests as minor as blood work, procedures, and hospitalizations. One study showed that the average physician has to make two or more calls to an HMO just to get treatment approved for each patient, approval that could be denied by the clerk at the other end of the line. Who's practicing medicine here?

In addition to managed health care, which includes health maintenance organizations (HMOs, where members pay a fixed fee for services), preferred providers organizations (PPOs, where members pay a set fee for services within the network, and more if they receive services from providers outside the network), and variations of these, there are private insurance plans; government programs such as Medicare, Medicaid, and other federal, state, and local plans; and no plans at all. Each of these has different qualifying requirements, precertification policies, and other rules. The instructions come in a thick booklet, written in such a way that you probably need a doctorate in order to understand them. Sometimes, even that isn't enough. Says one physician, "When I was applying for insurance payment, I, with an M.D., my wife, with a master's and the equivalent of a Ph.D., and my daughter, with a Ph.D., needed to rely on my son, who is a lawyer, to decipher the minutiae in the insurance coverage material and the details on the application forms." (It's been suggested, although not proven, that the writers of your insurance regulations also write VCR and computer software instructions.)

So who is benefitting from today's health insurance plans? It often isn't the physicians, who may have been required to sign a "gag clause" (now banned by at least six states), which prohibits them from discussing the treatment or medication they would have preferred to use had it been approved by the HMO or the risks the patient faces without the specific medication, test, or procedure. Recent federal legislation has prevented insurance companies from using gag clauses on federally insured patients.

It isn't the hospitals, which are forced to reduce staff to the minimum and supplement with less trained part-time workers, discharge patients even when their own medical staff knows it's too soon, and cut back on research and education funding. (Indeed, some of our most brilliant researchers are leaving major medical centers for lack of funding for their projects.)

It certainly isn't the patients, who, as Jerome P. Kassirer, M.D., so eloquently phrased it in an article in *The New England Journal of Medicine,* " . . . need to know that their physicians are not only at their side, but on their side."[1] We usually don't even realize that our doctor may have split allegiances, torn between remaining our advocate or remaining in practice, albeit with Big Brother

---

[1]*Kassirer, Jerome P., M.D., "Managed Care and the Morality of the Marketplace,"*
The New England Journal of Medicine *333, no. 1 (6 July 1995): 51.*

HMO ever watching. Furthermore, we may think we're properly covered . . . until we get sick. Then the fine print comes into focus: payment only for that which is "medically necessary" (who determines the criteria?), precertification for emergency treatment *not* resulting in hospitalization (how would you know before being treated that your chest pains were indigestion, not a coronary, or that your 45-minute nasal hemorrhage would finally clot?), and no pay for "investigational" treatments, which could include almost anything, subject to interpretation.

So who's benefitting? Could it be the top executives of the HMOs with salaries matching those of many professional basketball players? (In 1994, according to an article in *Newsday,* the cash and stock awards to the chiefs of the seven biggest for-profit HMOs averaged $7 million each.[2]) Could it be the stockholders, where "healthy" refers not to the patient subscribers, but to the stockholders' portfolios? Has medicine become merely dollar-driven with patients as products? We think so.

WHEN MORE IS LESS

The underlying policy for most managed care companies seems to be, "regardless how much the patient has paid in, let's limit what we pay out." Insurance is big business, you see, and the stockholders want great financial returns. They can realize this by controlling services covered. Managed-care organizations are practicing medicine without a license and we, the public, along with our government have permitted this to happen. The managed-care groups deny the charge, of course, pointing to the numerous M.D.s on their staff.

Nevertheless, they and their clerks (who really handle the majority of the calls and who do not hold medical degrees) are practicing mechanical medicine. These insurance companies have computed set fees for specific illnesses (called diagnostic-related

[2]Leon Eisenberg, "*Managed Health Care Needs a Watchdog,*" Newsday, 6 September 1995.

groupings or DRGs), mandating the allotted time one should spend in the hospital, ignoring the reality that each of us is an individual, with different healing abilities, ages, medical conditions, and personal circumstances. These faceless practioners can't possibly know that Mrs. Jadiwoski needs more time than the insurance-stipulated three days to recovery from her surgery. Why? Because when she gets home she has to care for both her husband, who has Alzheimer's disease, and a profoundly retarded child. Her personal physician knows it, though. But only if he or she is diligent and willing to be penalized for keeping a patient in the hospital longer may the doctor prevail—and then not without spending a great deal of time and effort in doing so. As one irate pediatrician confided, "I spend more time on the phone arguing with some high-school–educated clerk as to why I need to hospitalize a child with cancer or order a specific test for a baby with hepatitis than I do seeing patients. It's frustrating. I thought *I* was the one who had gone to medical school to practice medicine, not some clerk at an insurance company."

It's ironic. We, along with many others, feel we've thrown the baby out with the bathwater. By trying to control costs and keep doctors from running up added expense by ordering unnecessary tests and doing questionable procedures, we're denying them the right to order necessary important tests and perform procedures that may, in many cases, be lifesaving. We're permitting health insurance company staffs to manage (i.e., control) our medical care. It's managed economics, not managed care. Most health insurance plans reward physicians for undertreating patients whenever possible.

The health maintenance organizations call this more-for-less philosophy "financial incentives" for the physicians. Often it is achieved through a system called capitation, which means the HMO pays the physician a flat fee for each patient. If you don't get sick, the doctor keeps the entire amount; if you need medical care, however, the doctor is docked for specialists called in. The original purpose of this was to provide an incentive for doctors to keep their patients healthy. What it means in reality, however, is that the doctors get *more* money from the HMO for treating the patient *less;* the more he or she treats a patient, the less money in the doctor's pocket. Would you have your car repaired by a body shop that received more money for doing less work on your car?

MERRY-GO-ROUND MEDICINE

Many state and local governmental agencies, such as school boards, set their insurance coverage out for bids every two or three years. As with most bidding procedures, the lowest bid usually wins the lucrative account. This means that the employees who are affected often must switch their health-care provider every other year. As one teacher said angrily, "My kids have had three different pediatricians over the past five years. Just when the doctor gets to know my kids and their medical histories, the school system selects a new HMO."

It's like a merry-go-round. Sometimes you're riding high with a good selection of doctors from which to choose (although some of the best-known board-certified physicians may be dropped once people have become subscribers); the next time you may feel you've hit the bottom with a list of physicians you've never heard of. Often, you end up with no brass ring, just a handful of air.

Why is merry-go-round medicine so hazardous to your health? Because there's no continuity of care. Your primary physician has no chance to get to know you or your family or collect "a careful history [which] provides 70 to 80 percent of the information needed for most diagnoses."[3] Those with chronic medical conditions such as hemophilia, cancer, asthma, arthritis, and so on are at greatest risk because follow-up is more difficult every time there's a new HMO in the picture. In addition, your new primary care physician may not be aware if you've had a poor reaction to various forms of treatment or drugs.

[3] Leon Eisenberg, "Medicine—Molecular, Monetary, or More Than Both?" Journal of the American Medical Association 274, no. 4 (26 July 1995): 331.

Moreover, the majority of HMOs today use a formulary—a list of specifically approved pharmaceuticals from which your doctor can prescribe. That means that the medication you're taking may not be the exact one your doctor would have preferred or selected for you if he or she were free to choose. Sometimes it really doesn't matter which of two similar drugs is used; often, however, it matters greatly and with certain medical conditions could even trigger serious side effects. Many HMOs only cover drugs in standard dosages; if you need less because of other medical conditions, age, or previous reactions to the drugs, you may not be able to get the medication in the proper dosage for you (other than trying to chop a pill in half without slicing off the tip of your finger) even though the drug is manufactured in a smaller dosage and is available by the pharmaceutical distributor.

Not only does your hospitalization need to be approved by your HMO, but the tests and procedures prescribed by your physician require approval as well. If a specific test is denied by your HMO because it's too expensive or deemed experimental (even if it's done routinely in other hospitals), your doctor will have to substitute another that is approved, even if the latter may be more invasive, be less conclusive, and have troublesome side effects due to your other existing medical conditions.

Although many physicians for the past ten years have been using densitometer (bone density) studies to test patients for early osteoporosis so it could be treated promptly, insurance companies considered it experimental and denied reimbursement. Only those able to pay for the test out of pocket were able to benefit from it. Not until February 1996 did Medicare finally approve densitometer testing and the other insurance companies fell in line behind them.

What does that tell us? That insurance companies today establish what will exist as standard medical procedures and medical diagnostic testing. Valuable new (and often less invasive, less painful, and less potentially harmful) procedures will be withheld from patients who need them (sometimes with their lives depending on them) until the procedures become economically beneficial for the health insurance companies to cover them.

What can you do about it? Probably nothing because most of us never know we're getting second-choice medical care. We don't know about new drugs on the market or new procedures or diagnostic tests that lie waiting in the wings for their chance to show their stuff. If you do know, however, complain big-time, to anyone who will listen—the doctor, hospital, your HMO, the state insurance inspector, or your state's peer review organization (PRO). This latter organization is a federally funded group of practicing doctors and other health-care professionals who monitor the quality of care for Medicare patients. Check for your state's 1-800 number in your phone book or look for it in the American Hospital Association's *Guide to the Health Care Field,* available at your local library.

Contact the media, if necessary, to get heard. Write to your state legislator and Congress representatives. Many people in the cemetery today are there because they were denied a follow-up mammogram, state-of-the-art cancer treatment, specific medications or procedures, or even hospitalization. To paraphrase Hillel, "If you are not for yourself, who will be?" Certainly not your HMO.

REMEMBER DAVID AND GOLIATH

It may seem an overwhelming task—taking on the giant health insurance industry. But remember the story of David and Goliath. The little guy can overcome by using his (or her) wits. Let your slingshot be knowledge and the stone, your assertiveness. These suggestions may help you get the most out of your medical health plan:

1. If you haven't as yet selected a health plan, get information from surveys conducted by groups such as The National Committee for Quality Assurance (NCQA).

Call 1-800-839-6487 for their free Accreditation Status List, or write for their booklet on selecting a plan at: 2000 L Street, N.W., Suite 500, Washington, D.C. 20036. They also may be contacted at http://www.ncqa.org on the World Wide Web.

2. Take the list of health-care providers received from your HMO or PPO and show it to friends who are physicians, nurses, or other health-care professionals. Listen carefully to what they say (or do not say) about the doctors on that list. Ask others in the plan who they use and whether they're satisfied with their choice. Don't just pick a doctor because the office is nearby or because you've heard the name. Take time to select carefully as your primary care physician is the key to opening doors to the proper specialists, if and when you need them. Your life could depend on this choice.

3. Read everything the HMO sends you. You may not understand it all, but highlight the points you do and ask about those you don't.

4. Make friends with your primary care physician's office staff; these are the individuals who make the appointments and who often can give you excellent advice on how to work the system.

5. If you are choosing between various HMO or PPO plans, don't necessarily select the cheapest one. It could be a costly mistake. Often it's worth paying a little more in order to have the physician and hospital of your choice.

6. If your health insurance is through your place of employment, tell the person in charge of human resources if you're not happy with the service you're getting. Your complaint may be the one that finally convinces your boss it's time for a change.

7. Ask your physician which medications, tests, or procedures he or she would suggest regardless if the insurance covers it or not. It may be worth paying for it out of your pocket. Be aware, however, that your doctor may be subject to a gag clause and could be fired from the HMO for giving you the information you deserve (despite the doctor's vowing through the Hippocractic Oath that he or she would "prescribe for the good of my patients according to my ability and my judgment . . . ").

8. Ask your physician if he or she has signed a gag order. If you get a vague answer in return, the answer probably is yes.

9. Ask your physician if the way he or she is compensated by the HMO will, in any way, alter decisions made concerning choice of treatment, medication, and/or procedures for you. While the answer may be an automatic "no," by asking the question you remind the physician of the valued trust relationship implied between doctor and patient. (Some physicians we interviewed for this book reluctantly admitted that it did, in some cases, affect their decisions.)

10. If your "gate keeper" won't open the gate for you to see a specialist or have a specific diagnostic test or treatment, find another who will, even if you have to pay for it yourself. While you should be able to talk freely to your primary care physician and explain your concerns and reasons why you feel you should have further specialized care, many managed care plans pay bonuses to primary care doctors who spend less money on specialists for patient care. While your physician should be your advocate, you have to stand up for yourself. Don't be like the woman with

symptoms suggesting that she should have a colonoscopy to check for colon cancer. She timidly mentioned to her primary care physician that her brother had died of colon cancer. Wanting to contain costs and postpone what could possibly be an unnecessary diagnostic test, he said she probably had irritable bowel syndrome, gave her a tranquilizer, and told her to learn to relax. When her colon cancer was finally discovered, it had metastasized to her liver.

11. Go over your primary physician's head, if necessary, and challenge the HMO yourself. Ask whoever answers for the supervisor. (Everyone has one.) Don't take "no" for an answer. The informed patient is a threat to the health insurance industry. If your primary physician is on your side, so much the better. It's (sometimes) a winning combination.

12. If you're not satisfied with the treatment you've received from your managed-care organization, talk about it with others. You may not be the only unhappy subscriber. Remember, for them it's a business and too many lost subscribers can affect profits; for you and your family, it's your lives. Doesn't that make it worth fighting for?

13. Write to your state legislator or Congress representatives or contact the media.

The goal of staying well (and alive) can be greatly affected by the rules and regulations of your health-care provider. Just like the running of the bulls in Pamplona, you have to keep your head up, know where you're going, quickly deviate from the expected course when necessary, and not let them gore you in the back.

Conclusion

The most magnificent act a human being can perform is to save another's life. It is the ultimate act of benevolence and instills a spiritual feeling in the donor. The reason we wrote this book is to save lives. We pray that our experiences can give lifesaving abilities to the readers of this book. If we can save one life, then our ambitions will be achieved.

Dr. Blau:

I personally credit myself with having saved but one life in my thirty-five-year medical career. It was in my intern year at Montefiore Hospital in New York City. The emergency room was staffed by interns (now PGY-1) on a rotating basis. I was called to see a patient who was having a seizure because he was anoxic (suffering from lack of oxygen caused by pneumonia, asthma, emphysema, or a number of other problems). In this case, he was anoxic because his muscles of respiration—as a matter of fact, all his voluntary muscles— were paralyzed. They were paralyzed by the second most deadly toxin known to man, the tetanus toxin.

Alan Whitlow (as I shall call him to protect his privacy) had indeed acquired tetanus from the most innocuous of all cuts a few weeks before. Unfortunately, he was never given a tetanus toxoid inoculation as a child and therefore acquired tetanus. It was a rare disease even then because of almost universal inoculations during childhood.

As I examined Alan he could not speak. He had previously been seen by the psychiatrist who thought that the patient would *not speak. When I tried to open Alan's mouth, his jaw was locked. My God, I thought. It's lockjaw.*

"*He needs a trach,*" *I quickly screamed to the ER staff. I hope someone knows how to do a tracheostomy, I prayed. I had never done one before and had a vague impression of where the trachea was and more importantly, where to cut into it. Fortunately, an anesthesiology resident was present and exclaimed,* "*I'll do it.*"

I blessed him for knowing how to do it. In a few minutes I would "*see one,*" *as is the medical expression for the triad, 'see one, do one, teach one.' All too often in medicine that attitude prevails. After seeing Alan Whitlow's trachea entered, I would be* "*qualified*" *to do one in the future.*

Alan's care was now turned over to me. He was admitted from the ER on a respirator with a tracheostomy to "*my floor.*" *If he ran a fever, I was called—even if I were off duty. Eventually, he regained his ability to breathe, walk, and get out of bed. I was proud. I had saved his life and he knew it. But more importantly, I knew it, too. It gave us a special bond.*

I felt heady, almost divine. I knew that, as he recovered, it was all due to me and the care I was providing. All of his activities—his walking, talking, kissing his parents, and even his laughter—all of it was because of my medical care. I was so proud that I invited my wife to the ward to see my achievement. Upon seeing the ravages of six weeks of a tracheostomy and a 30-pound weight loss, my then pregnant wife fainted. For me, it was the best I ever felt in medicine in my life.

And when, ten years later, Alan was killed in cross fire during a robbery where he was an innocent bystander, I cried. His mother called to thank me for the ten extra years I had given her with her son. I cried again. So I guess that's one reason I wanted to write this book—to find Alan Whitlow again.

My experience as a hospitalized patient changed every aspect of my professional and emotional life. First and foremost, it made me a far more caring person. This has changed how I practice medicine. For the first time in my life, I enjoy the practice of medicine. Personal interaction with my patients at a level I never knew possible has given me tremendous satisfaction. I now know how many grandchildren every one of my patients has.

My experience as a patient has taught me even more than before that caution must be exercised before any medical decision is made. Even something as seemingly innocuous as having a blood test has its hazards because you can get an infection or hepatitis from a non-sterile needle. Also, the test results can give a false positive or negative, throwing you into treatment for something you may not have or no treatment for something you do. As of this writing, I encourage my male patients to have a PSA determination (testing for the presence of prostate cancer), but urge them to be aware that an elevated PSA determination is not synonymous with having a cancer of the prostate. Abnormal lab studies of any sort should always be re-tested, even if you have to pay for it yourself.

My fear is being in the "medical loop," that no-man's-land in clinical practice where something must be done because it makes sense and we have the know-how to do it. Going into the medical loop is the chain of events that occurs when an abnormality (often a false positive) is discovered. In the event that the patient refuses to follow prescribed therapy after discovering an abnormal blood test, he or she may feel guilty (especially if the loop path was correct) and the patient becomes ill.

I have two medical partners. One is an Orthodox Jew, who is blessed with inordinate skill, both as a physician and as a decision maker. He has refused to have a serum cholesterol test. After mine was discovered to be over 300 (years before my heart surgery), I spent years compulsively exercising, eating fake butter preparations that tasted like (and, indeed, may have been) Vaseline. I have figuratively seen a finger wagging back and forth in the sky if I ate a frankfurter. I have even done some paranoid, vicarious, imaginary calculations telling the world how many bacon-cheese omelets one had to eat before death was imminent.

My medical partner, on the other hand, hasn't spent one moment wasting his precious thoughts (and time) with such nonsense. His answer to runners, dieters, vegetarians, and eaters of Vaseline is one word, bershert. That word, the Hebrew word for "ordained" or "unchangeable," has survived for 10,000 years.

The next lesson that I learned from my near-death experience is that just going into a hospital as a patient is a death-defying act. Dying may be the worst thing that can happen to you; not necessarily the most painful, only the worst.

To go into a hospital for an elective procedure is a testimony to man's (and woman's) masochism. Once you are in the hospital, you must keep a constant vigil. You must always remember that there are people there who, without intending to, are in danger of killing you. They do this by their occasional lapse in the fragile chain that constitutes your care. Any seemingly minor error can result in your demise. That's why all hospitals have morgues.

So, knowing that you can be killed through an oversight or with the best intentions by some very skilled people, how can you stay out of the morgue? Begin by remembering that all of the people around you are capable of grievous error. (Being human means being fallible.) You must constantly be on guard against their errors.

I have personally found that there is no substitute for your own live-in advocate. Mine was my wife, who slept on a five-foot bench every night of my internment. If it were not *for her vigilant eye, I would be dead. It was she who diligently noted that one doctor was trying to expand my blood volume by giving me blood, while another was trying to reduce it with diuretics. In the presence of hypotension (extremely low blood pressure), the use of a diuretic can kill you. It was also my wife who discovered and reported to me that there was a staph epidemic on the ward.*

The most important thing a hospitalized patient can do is to bring in a relative or close friend, who will observe all and question everything being done *to the potential morgue inhabitant. Having such an advocate who is a spouse is one of the many benefits of a long marriage. (I have been married for thirty-eight years.)*

Also, I learned more about the insurance industry first-hand than I ever realized. If ever there was an argument for socialized medicine, it's the insurance industry itself. Managed care means managed economics. My insurance policy cost $12,000 a year. Despite the premium, the number-one priority of the insurance company is not *to pay the claim or to pay less of it than it costs. Words like "deductible," "co-pay," "reasonable charge," and "prevailing fee" are created by the insurance company to give you less than you thought you were going to get. The first letter I received upon leaving the hospital after my emergency surgery was that I was to be penalized because I did not let my insurance company know twenty-four hours prior to emergency surgery that I was going to need emergency surgery because the hospital ruptured my coronary artery! (Yes, if it weren't so serious, it would be the stuff of which sitcoms are made.)*

Now, theoretically, if I had known that they were going to rupture my coronary artery, perhaps I could have cancelled the entire procedure. That way it would have cost them nothing. Subsequent checks from the "wraparound" people (perhaps they call themselves "wraparound" because they never covered you), have never been for the amount submitted. Always less.

The vast amounts of money being made by the insurance industry on the backs of sick people is one of the great inequities of our society. It is unjust and immoral for people who are ill to be penalized in so many ways. Truly great societies will be remembered by the care they give to their most disadvantaged members.

The final lesson I learned from my canceled morgue appearance is the power of positive thinking, which my coauthor and I wholeheartedly subscribe to and practice. We believe that we are all potentially either victims or survivors. The victim passively permits all of the errors that can befall him or her in the hospital to occur. The victim believes that it's all in God's hands. While a good part of it is, it is you, who by action and control, can make a difference between surviving and dying. You must always assume that anything can go wrong and on an average day in an average hospital, it will.

The survivor, on the other hand, has succeeded in avoiding the morgue by taking those opportunities, not even seen by the victim, to question, to doubt, to be certain of the unwitting attempts by the entire hospital staff, to inadvertently get him or her into the morgue.

It's too simplistic to say that the best way to get out of the hospital alive is not to be admitted in the first place. There are many times when we must be in the hospital in order to receive proper care and treatment. But along with our toothbrush and slippers, we need to take a sense of responsibility with us.

We cannot be passive in the hospital, but must take an active part in our treatment and our care. It cannot deteriorate into a "them and us" mentality, with the doctors or the hospital the bad guys. Restrictions placed on both the physician and the institution by health insurance companies have made it necessary for hospitals to enlist the patients' cooperation and support. In some cases, these collaborations have created positive change. One such example is the so-called "drive-by-deliveries" triggered by the insurance companies' insistence on sending newborns and their moms home less than twenty-four hours after delivery. Complaints by obstetricians, pediatricians, hospitals, and parents alike turned to teamwork between physicians, patients, and the hospitals. Experts for the Centers for Disease Control and Prevention, the American Medical Association, the American College of Obstetricians and Gynecologists, and the American Pediatric Association all threw in their support. All these efforts forced Congress to pass legislation stipulating that it was a proper decision to be made between patient and doctor.

Yet insurance HMOs have forced hospitals to continue to tighten their belts and staff reductions have made it difficult for most medical institutions to give the same attentive care as in previous times. Part-time employees are brought in when needed, so there is less cohesiveness on the floors. For this and other reasons, we feel it is imperative for patients to have someone with them at all times—especially, but not restricted to children, the elderly, and those unable to speak up for themselves—in order to monitor the medications, answer questions, and, most importantly, to ask questions.

Obviously, it is often impractical for one caregiver to remain in the hospital with a patient at all times. However, other family members, friends, and support teams from churches or synagogues can be educated to serve as the active participant in the patient's care. Information, medicines, allergies, and other complete background material can be written down and passed along to those who watch, not only to be on the lookout for errors, but also to support the overburdened hospital staff, most of whom want to give care, concern, and caution, but are under stress to do more with less help.

How can we get out of the hospital alive? By becoming truly informed, remaining alert and assertive, asking questions, becoming an active part of your health-care team, with a little bit of luck, and God's will.

Medical Terms
You Should Know

A lthough all professions have their own jargon, the medical field—followed closely by the legal field—tends to win in the race to most confuse those not in its membership. Its use of acronyms and tongue-twisting terms seems to be based on a need to make things appear more mystical, which is strange considering the profession is steeped in a scientific tradition. Use this listing as your "crib sheet" to help you understand what the doctors and nurses are talking about and saying about you.

Acuity: Sharpness, as in your vision or hearing.

Acute: Sharp as in pain or of sudden onset.

Afebrile: Without fever.

Analgesic: A medication or procedure, such as acupuncture, to stop or reduce pain.

Angiography: A test in which a solution that can be seen on X rays is injected into blood vessels in order to check for potential blockages. The photos resulting from this procedure are known as **angiograms.**

Angioplasty: A surgical procedure in which a small flexible tube (catheter) with a balloon at one end is fed into a section of an artery that has narrowed because of disease. The balloon is then inflated in order to open the artery.

Anticoagulent: A drug used to prevent blood clot formation.

Antiemetic: A drug used to prevent or reduce nausea or vomiting.

Arrhythmias: Variations in the normal heartbeat.

Arthrocentesis: The removal of joint fluid.

Arthroscopy: Examination of the inside of a joint by using a thin optical instrument.

Ascites: Fluid in the abdominal cavity caused by disease of the heart, liver, kidney, or blood.

Asepsis: Absence of infection.

Aspiration: A procedure in which fluid is drained from a cyst or body cavity by a needle and syringe, or needle and Vacutainer tube.

Asymptomatic: Without symptoms.

Ataxia: Lack of motor coordination due to nerve or brain injury, disease, or medication.

Atheroma: Fatty tissue that adheres to the walls of a person's arteries, narrowing the passage.

Barium: A chemical, barium sulfate, which shows up on X rays. If inserted rectally, it is called a **barium enema** and reveals masses on the lining of the colon and rectum. If mixed with flavored fluids and filmed as first swallowed, it is called a **barium swallow,** and reveals the esophagus; if filmed as the liquid goes down the digestive tract, it is called a **barium meal,** and reveals the entire digestive tract. These procedures are used to detect diseases of the gastrointestinal system.

Benign: This term means "not malignant." A benign growth is one that is not cancerous and will not spread.

Biopsy: A surgical procedure in which a small sampling of bodily tissue is removed to study under a microscope in order to determine if it is malignant.

Blood poisoning: Also known as **septicemia.** It is caused by bacteria invading the bloodstream and multiplying or by nonbacterial toxins. Bacteremia is bacteria in the bloodstream; septicemia is the products of bacteria in the bloodstream.

Bone marrow: The innermost area of bone that is the precursor of blood cells.

Bougenage: The dilatation of a tubular organ (such as esophagus).

Bronchoscopy: A procedure in which a thin flexible instrument, called a **bronchoscope,** is passed down the throat in order to study the air passages of the lungs.

Bypass: Diversion of substances, usually fluids (such as blood, urine, spinal fluid, feces), sometimes referred to as shunting. Most commonly associated with coronary artery bypass.

CABG: Coronary artery bypass graft.

Carcinoma: A malignant growth.

Cardiac catheterization: A procedure carried out under local anesthetic in which a flexible tube is fed into a blood vessel and into the heart in order to check the functioning of the heart.

Cardiocentesis: The aspiration of fluid from around the heart.

Carotid arteriograms: A procedure in which a dye is injected into the carotid artery in the neck. X rays are taken as the dye moves through the blood vessels into the brain. This procedure is used as a diagnostic tool when someone has suffered a stroke or other abnormalities.

CAT scan: Also known as **computerized axial tomography.** This is a painless diagnostic procedure in which multiple X-ray pictures are taken of the head or other part of the body and processed by a computer, which illustrates details in slice-like views.

Colonoscopy: A procedure in which a lighted flexible tube is inserted into the rectum to the colon, allowing the physician to visually examine the colon.

Contracture: The shortening of a muscle, tendon, scar tissue, or any structure caused by injury, disease, birth defect, or disuse.

Coronary arteriography: Angiography of the heart muscle done during the cardiac cath procedure. The pictures, called **coronary**

arteriograms, reveal areas and types of problems in the heart and blood vessels.

Cyanosis: A blue discoloration of the lips or skin due to blood with unoxygenated hemoglobin, which often means that the body is not getting enough oxygen.

Cystoscope: A lighted tube and viewing lens inserted through the urethra in order to visually examine the interior of the bladder.

Diastolic: The lower number on a blood pressure reading, which measures the heart cycle pressure when the **ventricles,** the lower chambers, are relaxed.

DRGs: Stands for Diagnostic Related Groups. It refers to an insurance creation in which hospitals are reimbursed for treatment based on a fixed, predetermined amount arrived at by figuring the average cost for that procedure.

Dysuria: Painful or difficult urination.

Echocardiography: A painless procedure in which the heart structure is examined by ultrasound waves. The findings are recorded graphically, called an **echogram.**

Endoscope: A tube-like instrument, often flexible, with a light and eyepiece, inserted in a bodily opening to view, photograph, and at times, biopsy, interior tissue. The procedure is called an **endoscopy.**

Epistaxis: Nosebleed.

Fibrillation: The abnormal rapid vibration of the heart muscle far in excess of the heart's normal rhythmical contractions.

Hematoma: A swelling filled with blood.

Intravenous infusion: Another term for an IV drip, in which medications, saline, vitamins, or other liquids are dripped from a bag, held by an elevated holder, into the body through a tube inserted into a vein.

Intravenous pyelography: Also referred to as IVP, this procedure is used to examine the urinary system. A special dye that shows up on X rays is injected into a vein.

Kidney biopsy: The removal of a small section of a kidney for diagnostic testing.

Lumbar puncture: Also known as a **spinal tap,** this procedure is used to diagnose injuries and diseases of the nervous system. Under a local anesthetic, a needle is inserted between the vertebrae at the base of the spine. A small amount of cerebrospinal fluid is removed for study.

Magnetic resonance imaging: Also known as an **MRI.** A magnetic imaging technique in which a scanning device using a magnetic field and radiofrequency energy is used to study bone, ligaments, tumors, soft tissues, and so on.

Malignant: A cancerous tumor or condition.

Meninges: The membranes covering the spinal cord and brain. If these become swollen—by injury or infection—the person may have severe headaches, stiff neck, vomiting, and fever.

Morbidity: The state of being ill.

Mycoplasma: A microorganism that causes, among other things, a respiratory infection known as **atypical pneumonia.** It is resistant to penicillin, but reacts to other antibiotics.

Myelography: An X-ray procedure in which a solution is injected into the spinal canal in order to study the spinal cord.

Nasogastric tube: A tube passed through the nose, down the throat, and into the stomach. It is used both for providing nourishment and for draining away digestive juices.

Needle biopsy: A sample of body tissue or fluid withdrawn by a syringe.

Nephrosis: Malfunctioning of the kidneys.

Nosocomial infection: An infection picked up in the hospital.

NPO: Nothing by mouth.

Occult: Hidden, as blood in stool that is not visible to the naked eye.

Paracentesis: A procedure in which fluid is withdrawn from a part of the body (usually the abdominal cavity) by a syringe for diagnostic or therapeutic purposes.

Parenteral nutrition: Nutritional substances delivered by any route other than orally.

Peritoneum: The abdominal lining.

Photophobia: Sensitivity to light.

Positron Emission Tomography: Also known as **PET.** A procedure used to study biochemical activity in the brain using radioactive isotopes.

Proctoscopy: Examining the anus and rectum through the use of a lighted scope with a magnifier eyepiece.

Proctosigmoidoscopy: Examining the rectum and sigmoid colon with a flexible lighted scope that penetrates further into the colon.

Remission: A period of time during which there is no sign of a previous disease.

Sepsis: Poisoning of body cells through infection or toxin.

Staphylococcus: A specific type of bacteria that can cause serious infection.

Status asthmaticus: Serious form of asthma that does not respond to usual treatment.

Stenosis: A narrowing, such as in a blood vessel, the spinal column, or heart valve openings.

Streptococcus: A specific type of bacteria responsible for strep throat, rheumatic fever, scarlet fever, and other diseases.

Syncope: Fainting.

Systolic: The first of two numbers given when blood pressure is taken. It refers to the period when the heart ventricles contract and blood is pumped into the arteries.

Tachycardia: An abnormally rapid heartbeat.

Tetany: Muscle cramps and spasms occasionally caused by lack of adequate calcium or magnesium, or by hyperventilation.

Thoracentesis: The aspiration of fluid in the chest.

Thrombus: A blood clot. If the clot breaks away, it is called an **emboli** or **embolism.**

Transient ischemic attack: Often called a **TIA** or "a little stroke." It is a temporary brain phenomenon triggered by a blockage or spasm of a cerebral artery.

Upper gastrointestinal series: Also known as **Upper GI.** These are diagnostic tests of the esophagus, stomach, and duodenum in which a barium drink is swallowed and its progress noted through the use of a fluoroscope and X ray.

APPENDIX B

Suggested Reading

Benson, Herbert, M.D., with Marge Stark. *Timeless Healing: The Power and Biology of Belief.* New York: Scribner, 1996.

Berger, Stuart M., M.D. *What Your Doctor Didn't Learn in Medical School.* New York: William Morrow, 1988.

Cousins, Norman. *Anatomy of an Illness as Perceived by the Patient.* New York: Norton, 1979.

———. *Head First: The Biology of Hope and the Healing Power of the Human Spirit.* New York: Penguin Books, 1989.

Graedon, Joe and Teresa Graedon, Ph.D. *The People's Guide to Deadly Drug Interactions.* New York: St. Martin's Press, 1995.

Heymann, Sally Jo. *Equal Partners.* Boston: Little Brown, 1995.

Horowitz, Lawrence, M.D. *Taking Charge of Your Medical Fate.* New York: Random House, 1988.

Inlander, Charles, Lowell Levin, and Ed Weiner. *Medicine on Trial.* New York: Prentice-Hall, 1988.

Inlander, Charles B. and Ed Weiner. *Take This Book to the Hospital with You.* Avenel, NJ: Wings Books, 1993.

Konner, Melvin, M.D. *Medicine at the Crossroads*. New York: Pantheon Books, 1993.

Locke, Steven, M.D., and Douglas Colligan. *The Healer Within*. New York: Dutton, 1986.

McCall, Timothy B., M.D. *Examining Your Doctor*. New York: Carol Publishing Group, 1995.

McCann, Karen Keating. *Take Charge of Your Hospital Stay*. New York: Insight Books, 1994.

Maurer, Janet M., M.D. *How to Talk to Your Doctor*. New York: Simon & Schuster, 1986.

Moyers, Bill. *Healing and the Mind*. New York: Doubleday, 1993.

Podell, Richard N., M.D., and William Proctor. *When Your Doctor Doesn't Know Best*. New York: Simon & Schuster, 1995.

Shimberg, Elaine Fantle. *Strokes: What Families Should Know*. New York: Ballantine Books, 1990.

Siegel, Bernie S. *Love, Medicine & Miracles*. New York: Harper Perennial, 1986.

————. *Peace, Love & Healing*. New York: Harper & Row, 1989.

Smith, Wesley J. *The Doctor Book: A Nuts and Bolts Guide to Patient Power*. Los Angeles: Price Stern Sloan, 1987.

Vickery, Donald M., M.D. *Taking Part: The Consumer's Guide to the Hospital*. New York: Center for Corporate Health, 1986, 1991.

Youngson, Robert, M.D. *The Surgery Book*. New York: Diagram Visual Information, 1993.

Index

A

Abductions of infants, 78,
  79–84
Achterberg, Jeanne, 176
Admitting office, 11, 24–28
Advanced directive, 23,
  114–15
Alcohol, 24, 97,
  112–13, 151
Allergies, 22, 71
  diagnostic procedures and,
    119, 125
  to foods, 75, 92
  to medications, 21, 25,
    71, 183
American Academy of
  Pediatrics, 27
American Board of
  Emergency
  Medicine, 13
American College
  of Emergency
  Physicians, 14, 15, 19
American College of
  Surgeons' Committee
  on Trauma, 12
American Hospital Asso-
  ciation (AHA), 8, 99
Amniocentesis, 119–20
Anatomy of an Illness
  (Cousins), 122–23,
  172, 176
Anesthesia, 113, 160
  adverse reactions to,
    151, 153
  breathing exercises
    and, 180
  for children, 154–55
  cortisone and, 153

epidural, 152, 153
informed consent for, 110
local, 152–53
regional, 153
Anesthesiologists, 46,
  149–58, 160
  medical history and,
    150–52, 153
  nurse anesthetists, 46,
    149, 157–58
  pain control and, 155–57
Angiography, 127
Angioplasty, 128
Anthropologist on Mars, An
  (Sacks), 179
Antibiotics, 55, 62–63
Antidepressants, 21, 69, 93
Arthroscopy, 128
Attacks and rapes, 78,
  84–86
Autologous transfusion,
  66, 75

B

Babies, abduction of,
  78, 79–84
Barium, 125, 132
Bedard, Larry, 14
Benson, Herbert, 175–76,
  179, 185
Biopsy, 128
Blood tests, 50, 129–30
Blood transfusions, 65–66,
  71, 75
Bone density studies, 197
Breathing, 180–81
Breckenridge, Joan, 189
Bronchoscopy, 128

C

Campbell, Douglas A., 91
Campbell, Sylvia, 185
Canter, Murray, 152
Cardiac catheterization, 130
Carotid arteriograms, 129
CAT (computerized axial
  tomography) scan, 129
CBC (complete blood
  count) test, 129–30
Certified registered nurse
  anesthetists (CRNAs),
  46, 157–58
Cesarean section, 138, 140
Chase, Scott M., 36
Children, 24, 30, 127
  anesthesiologists and,
    154–55
  pain control for, 181–82
  pediatric specialists for,
    18–19, 46, 154–55
  play therapists and, 51–52
  private rooms for, 27–28
Choking, 94–95
Chopra, Deepak, 172,
  176, 177
Clergy, 53
Colonoscopy, 125–26,
  130–31
Colon surgeons, 45
Communication
  doctors' skills in, 38–40, 44
  language and other
    difficulties in, 19,
    23, 181
  truthfulness and
    completeness in,
    22–23, 24, 25,
    112–13, 150–51